THE VIELS' BEAUTY BIBLE

*Look and feel
fabulous with or without
cosmetic surgery.*

DR ROBERTO AND DR MAURIZIO VIEL

Cosmetic surgeons to the stars

HODDER
MOBIUS

First published in Great Britain in 2006
by Hodder & Stoughton
A division of Hodder Headline

The right of Dr Roberto and Dr Maurizio
Viel to be identified as the Authors of the
Work has been asserted by them in
accordance with the Copyright,
Designs and Patents Act 1988.

A Mobius Book

1

A CIP catalogue record for this title is
available from the British Library

ISBN 978 0 340 92367 2
ISBN 0 340 92367 9

Designed by Ash
Illustrations © Yoko

Colour reproduction by Dot Gradations Ltd
Printed and bound in Great Britain
by CPI Bath Press

Hodder Headline's policy is to use papers
that are natural, renewable and recyclable
products and made from wood grown in
sustainable forests. The logging and
manufacturing processes are expected to
conform to the environmental regulations
of the country of origin.

Hodder & Stoughton Ltd
A division of Hodder Headline
338 Euston Road
London NW1 3BH

To Luigi Viel … our beloved father and inspiration

There have been so many people whom we have met over the course of our lives, people who have been a source of help, inspiration and advice. We want to thank all of you for everything you have given us and if we have forgotten anyone, we apologise.

We would first of all like to thank our Mama Giuseppina, Uncle Mario and all of our beloved family. Roberto's wife Laura, and his two children Beatrice and Alberto and Maurizio's girlfriend Romana. Thanks to you all for your love and support in all we do.

We extend our thanks, admiration and appreciation to Jane Alexander, for her patience!! and for helping us to write this book; and of course to Rowena, Helen, Fenella and everyone at Hodder for believing in us and for commissioning *The Beauty Bible*. To our book agent David Smith and to our television agent Philip Chard.

We would like to give a special thanks to Kate, Liz, Sandra, Katya and everyone at The London Centre for Aesthetic Surgery for all of your constant hard work and to all of our other colleagues for your help, support, advice and feedback. Thank you also to our long time friends and colleagues Dr Franz Noorman Van der Dussen and Dr Massamiliano Marcelino.

Thank you to Robert Montague and everyone at RKM Public Relations Ltd who look after our press and publicity and who drove this project forward. Thank you for all of your support, effort and good work over the years and long may we continue together.

Our final thanks go to all of the many patients we have had over the years, thank you to you all.

"Grazie tutti per ogni cosa, Baci e abbracci … Ciao"
Roberto e Maurizio

Contents

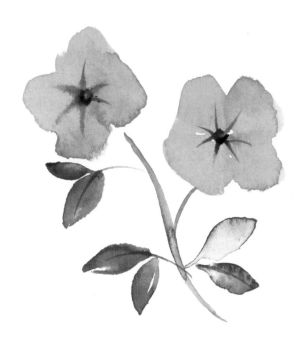

Introduction

Let's be honest, we all want to look younger and feel better. We've all stood in front of the mirror and gently pulled up a little skin to reveal a fresher face. We've all looked at those 'before and after' shots and wondered how our own faces and bodies might look if we gave nature a helping hand. There isn't a woman alive who hasn't dreamed of having a bit more 'up top' or a little less down below; who hasn't fantasised about a pert new nose or a trim pair of thighs. Between us, we have helped literally thousands of women look younger and feel fantastic – both with and without the use of surgery. We know every trick in the book (and then a few) to make you look and feel the best you ever have, however old you might be in biological years.

Don't for one moment think you're the only one who dreams of some radical rejuvenation. Nine out of ten Britons say they would like to change something about their appearance. A quarter of the population would be up for a 'dramatic overhaul'. The number of cosmetic procedures performed more than doubled last year. More and more people are having cosmetic surgery and the procedures are becoming more sophisticated, more subtle, and more safe. Even if you don't fancy going under the knife, there are still masses of things you can do that will make a truly astonishing difference to your appearance. The whole field of cosmetic surgery is changing. No longer are we surgeons merely nip and tuck scalpel-wielders – we now offer total rejuvenation, using the latest research in nutrition, exercise, supplements and hormone therapy, alongside an ever increasing number of totally non-invasive procedures.

It's a hugely exciting time: never before have we been given the chance to stay looking so young for so long. Don't you owe it to yourself to be the very best you can?

Don't think this new rejuvenation therapy is just for celebrities or the super-rich either. This book is for everyone who ever wanted to look and feel more gorgeous. Why *shouldn't* you look the best you can? Who *wouldn't* want to look their very best? Giving in and ageing gracefully? We don't think so.

It's easy to criticise our business, claiming it's fuelled by nothing more than vanity and insecurity. We disagree. Like it or not, our confidence is partly (and largely) defined by the way we look; our self-esteem is inextricably bound up with our image. If you look better on the outside, you automatically feel better on the inside and suddenly the world seems like a much nicer place. Rejuvenation is *not* just about vanity. We are quite emphatic about that. Time after time we have seen the same amazing thing happen. Patients tell us their entire lives have changed following our work. We have seen alterations (often quite minor shifts) in appearance give an exponential boost to self-esteem and confidence. Our patients frequently tell us that our techniques have super-charged their careers or their love lives; boosted their chances of promotion or helped them get hitched!

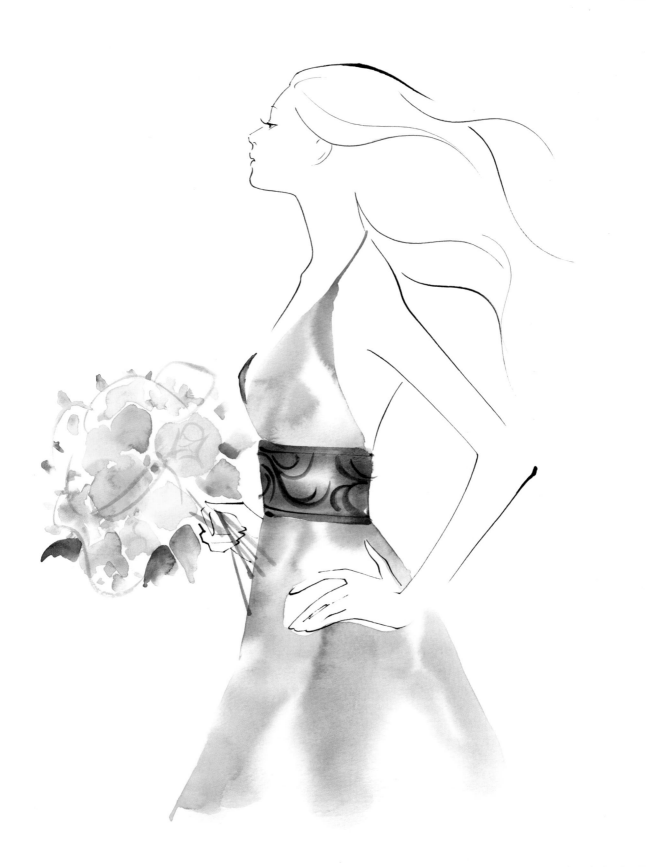

It's not just nip and tuck

We have been performing cosmetic surgery for the past twenty years. Between us we carry out around a thousand procedures per year and we have pioneered many of the newest, more exciting procedures in the business. We firmly believe cosmetic surgery is a tool for good, a highly effective tool of transformation. However we don't always reach for the scalpel. Over the years we have discovered that, for the very best results, you need to take a holistic approach. Unlike many cosmetic surgeons, we build up a long-term relationship with our patients, helping them overhaul their entire lives, from the foods they eat to the way they stand; we look at their relationships, their work, their self-image and their deep psyches. Sometimes we don't even recommend surgery at all – or not at that particular time. We counsel our patients so they can make the right choices, whether that be radical surgery, non-invasive procedures or even no surgery at all. Looking good isn't just about going under the knife: we will scrutinise every aspect of your well-being and help you choose the most effective ways to look your very best. There are absolutely hordes of things you can do that will make you look and feel better, without even a whiff of anaesthetic. A-list beauties know the power of diet, exercise and posture. They're wise to the myriad wonder creams and non-invasive techniques that make skin look fresh and young, that slim and tone bodies. We'll let you in on all the secrets.

Above all, we would like to point out that cosmetic surgery is not about an unrealistic quest for perfection: it's about improving what you have, about making the very best of yourself. We will be quite blunt about what cosmetic surgery *can't* do – and what it *shouldn't* do.

Helping you make the best possible choice

We hope that this book will give you all the information you could possibly need to make the very best possible decision for yourself. While the majority of cosmetic surgeons are ethical, responsible professionals, this is still an industry that needs much more regulation. Although the situation is not as bad as it was in the past (when any doctor could set themselves up as a cosmetic surgeon without any specialist training) it still – or so we feel – does not have enough controls. So you do need to be wary, and you do need to do your homework. We will give you the tools you need to be able to discern a good clinic and a good surgeon from a less scrupulous one. Cosmetic surgery is expensive and we don't want you to waste your money, or have a less than ideal result.

If you do decide to go for surgery we will help you make up your mind what you really need, and why. Not everyone is a good candidate for surgery and not every procedure is ideal for everyone. We'll help you make smart decisions. We'll also be encouraging you to alter your view of surgeons. In the past you would barely even see your surgeon. If you went into hospital for an operation, they might drop by your bed for a brief consult, but that would probably be the only (conscious) time you'd be in the same room. We believe, however, that you should treat your cosmetic surgeon in the same way you treat your GP – as someone with whom you have a long-term, close, trusting relationship. A good surgeon will not want you to have all your surgery at once (although there are certain procedures that can work well when conducted at the same time).

Your surgeon will aim for subtle results, performing procedures over the years to keep you looking and feeling your very best. In the past, people would delay the process until the last possible moment, and then go for drastic lifts and tucks. Now we much prefer to start as early as possible, using preventative treatment and non-invasive procedures so that major invasive surgery can often be avoided for much, much longer.

Love yourself. Treat your body as the most wonderful machine in the universe – respect it.

Live life to the full

Nobody's perfect and we don't peddle perfection. But if you can iron out your flaws, why on earth not? Is it really a virtue to traipse through life feeling less than confident, less than happy, when you could do something about it? Are you really going to lie on your deathbed and feel guilty about having had cosmetic surgery? We can't see it, personally. However you might well regret that you didn't take the chance to live your life to the full. You might regret that you didn't grab life with both hands and get the most out of it. You might regret all the opportunities you lost or didn't have the nerve to grasp, because you simply didn't have the confidence. Because, bottom line, beautification and rejuvenation are really all about self-esteem and confidence. That is why we are such passionate advocates of cosmetic surgery, of anti-ageing techniques, of beauty enhancements. Our job gives us huge and lasting satisfaction because we have the ability to – quite literally – change people's lives. If you can change a face, or a body, and help the way someone feels about themselves, that can't be wrong. In the past, medicine was purely for saving lives. Now it's for enhancing lives.

We live in exciting times. No previous generation has had this opportunity to reinvent themselves throughout their lives. No longer do we have to accept meekly what nature gave us and make the most of it. Life is wonderful and you owe it to yourself to make the very most of it. This book can help you. As our Roman forebears said, '*Carpe diem*' – so go on, seize the day!

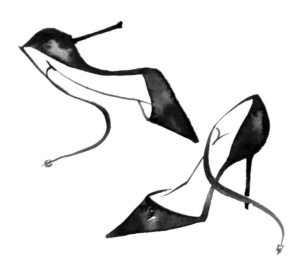

CHAPTER ONE

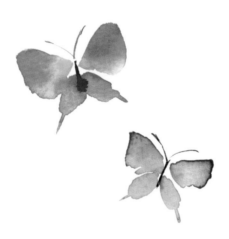

What is beauty –
and why is it so important?

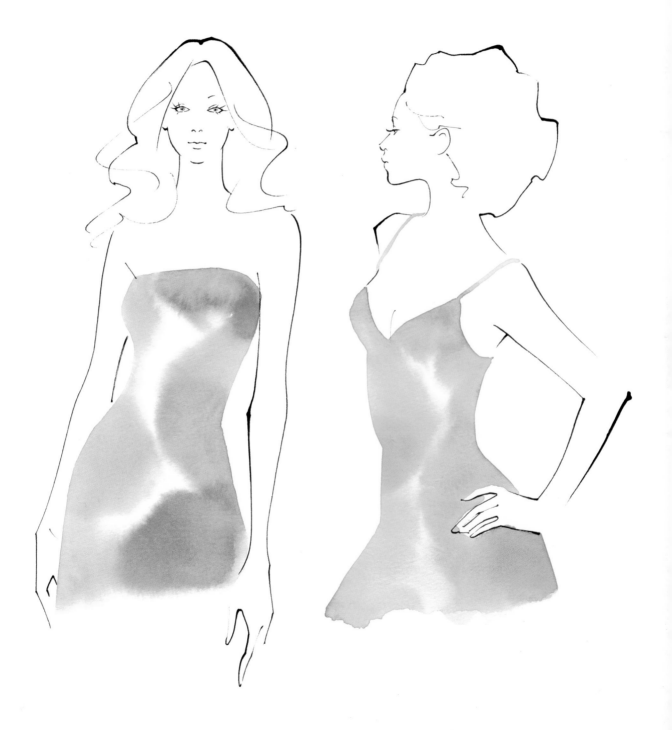

We believe wholeheartedly in beauty. Well, we are Italians after all! In fact, we'd go further and say that beauty is one of the most important aspects of life. Beauty is not confined to a lovely face but extends to everything in life, whether it be a beach, a mountain, a building, a body. For us, the key elements are harmony and proportion. When you look at something or someone, you want to see something harmonious, something lovely. You don't want to look at something that sticks out, that isn't in proportion, that doesn't have harmony. For something to be beautiful, it is absolutely essential that it is pleasing to the eye. When that happens, it's akin to love. It gives you, the viewer, a sense of well-being, a feeling of peace and tranquillity. When people fall in love, they are linked by chemistry – desire triggers a part of the brain which in turn sends out neurochemicals that make you feel good. A similar mechanism comes into play when we look on beauty, be it in a person or a landscape or a stunning piece of architecture. The brain sends out feelings of intense happiness.

To our minds, there is no such thing as a 'perfect' nose or a 'perfect' pair of eyes – a technically imperfect nose or eyes can be perfect in a particular face. Beauty, we feel, is intensely, passionately personal. What we consider beautiful, you might not see, and vice versa. You simply cannot turn beauty into a mathematical equation. In the textbooks for plastic surgery there are angles, and lines and shapes that are considered ideal, but if you apply them to a real living face or body, they won't necessarily work. They might not go with the colour of your hair, or your skin tone, or your height. The perfect eyes and nose are those that work together: harmony.

Way back in the second century, the philosopher Galen said: 'Beauty does not lie in the individual elements, but in the harmonious proportion of the parts, in the proportion of one finger in relation to another, of all the fingers to the whole hand, of the rest of the hand to the wrist, of this last to the forearm, of the forearm to the whole arm, and finally of all the parts to all the others.' We couldn't agree more.

Beauty shifts too, according to time and place. As our countryman Umberto Eco says in his intriguing book, *On Beauty*: 'Beauty has never been absolute and immutable but has taken on different aspects depending on the historical period and the country.' You only need to walk through a large art gallery to see the truth in that. While faces don't change so much, bodies certainly do. The medieval artists portrayed slim, small-breasted women in stark contrast to the voluptuous folds of flesh in which Rubens revelled. In some countries, fat is still considered beautiful and the flabbier you are, the more attractive you are seen to be.

The beauty trap

However unfair it may seem, we are judged by the way we look. Think back to the playground, when you were a child. Ten to one you will remember the 'fat one' or 'the one with the sticking-out ears' or 'the one who was as flat as a pancake'. Children are cruel and many people remain scarred for life by the thoughtless jibes of their playmates. However it's not just children who judge us on the size of our legs or the shape of our chin. Research shows quite clearly that adults also make huge value judgements based only on the way someone looks. For example:

- Fat people are greedy and lazy.

- People with flat squashed noses are looking for a fight.

- People with 'jug' ears are stupid.

- Men with small chins are weak.

- You can't trust a person whose eyes are close together.

The obverse is also true. People instinctively attribute positive personality characteristics to people who are physically attractive. We prefer to date and mate with attractive people. We may swear blind that 'looks don't matter' or that we would much prefer our partners and associates to have a good sense of humour or an incisive brain rather than a pretty face, but it's simply not true. Research shows that the single factor that will produce satisfaction with a blind date, for example, is facial attractiveness (and that goes for both men and women).

You might think this 'beauty-ism' only affects us when we're looking for a mate, but that just isn't so. Scientists have found that attractiveness affects virtually every part of our lives. We choose employees as much for the way they look as the way they work. We even vote for beauty, picking our political leaders not just on their economic and social policies, but on the shape of their faces and the width of their eyes. Scientists call this the 'attractiveness halo effect' or the 'beauty is good stereotype'. If you fancy a life of crime make sure you're good-looking, as attractive criminals get lighter sentences than their uglier counterparts. And, baby, you'd better score high in the cute factor, as (rather shockingly) mothers bond more readily with attractive infants and premature babies with appealing looks receive more care than their pug-faced peers. Incredible though it may seem, in today's supposedly enlightened society, people who are considered to have nice looks have been shown, in study after study, to get a nicer deal, a better shot at life.

What *is* beauty, after all?

While beauty is very individual, research shows that there are some aspects of beauty that remain constant. Science has found that there are certain factors that combine to make up as near as we can come to a 'perfect' face. From the moment we are born, we learn to recognise beauty. Even very young babies would rather look at attractive faces than ugly ones. And the notion of what constitutes an attractive face is, curiously, exactly the same for small babies as it is for fully grown adults. While the desirability of body shapes changes over the years (according to fashion or according to culture), a pretty face seems to remain relatively constant. Research has even shown that people from very different cultures are still attracted to the same types of faces, so it appears that there is something fundamental about a large part of our concept of beauty. So, what is it we look for in a face?

1   **Symmetry:** we like balanced faces. There are two different explanations for this.

- We are attracted to people with symmetrical faces because they would make good mates. This follows because symmetry gives us an indication of how healthy we are. If we are strong, with a healthy immune system and no genetic defects, we will develop symmetrical faces in the womb. If we are weaker, we are more likely to suffer disease or infection during our development and so small imperfections (asymmetries) can occur. Therefore having a symmetrical face implies that we have a strong immune system, able to fight off illness. This is obviously a good thing when you are looking for a mate as it suggests good genes and a capacity to protect and care for the family.

- We are 'hard-wired' in such a way that it's easier for us to make sense of symmetrical stimuli than it is to process asymmetrical stimuli. So it's simply easier for us to look at symmetrical faces (it's also been shown that we prefer symmetry in art and sculpture).

Of course, these explanations could well be part and parcel of the same thing: we find it easier to look at symmetry so we are automatically attracted to people with good genes and a healthy immune system. Whatever, it doesn't really matter – the point is a symmetrical face is an attractive face.

2   **Exaggeration:** scientists used to think we liked average safe faces, but that's not quite true. We like a certain amount of exaggeration in our facial characteristics. This varies markedly between the sexes. Large lips and eyes are seen as attractive in women while large noses and chins are not. Men, however, are often deemed attractive with larger noses, pronounced brow ridges and 'strong' jaws. Once again, it seems to come down to indications of a person's reproductive capabilities: those people with the most exaggerated sex-typical traits are perceived as being the healthiest and most fertile. What's fascinating is that, while men

universally prefer very 'feminine' faces in women, women don't always go for the most 'masculine'-faced men. Scientists think this is because women are not only looking for a potential sperm-donor with strong genes but also for a good long-term mate, someone with the ability to be a good, caring father (and feminine features imply a good carer).

3   Youthful features: we are attracted to youthful faces, time and time again. Once more, this is perceived as a biological safety net. Young women, whether we like it or not, tend to be more fertile and have healthier babies. Hence society's obsession with ultra-youthful girl-women. Men have a little more leeway here as a man can effectively father a child right into old age. However women are biologically wired to seek a mate who can not only father her child but provide for and protect that child. Hence very youthful features are not so attractive in men, but neither are those that imply old age or infirmity. Women look for features that indicate a man in his prime, physically, sexually and financially. Unfair? Certainly. But who said nature is fair?

4   Open, happy faces: it's not just *how* we look, it's the way we look. Facial expressions, or perceived expressions, are vital too. It's all pretty obvious: we prefer people who smile to people who don't. We like people who look directly at us rather than those who appear to be glancing away from us. Someone's facial expression indicates how they are feeling towards you, and their gaze indicates how much attention they are giving you. How interested a person is in you seems as important as how attractive they may be. We are also hard-wired to detect if there is any potential danger around. So we will notice, and be repelled by, a face that appears angry, particularly if that person is gazing directly at us. Equally, a face that appears shifty, with an avoidance of eye contact, may send off warning signals.

This is all fascinating, but does it really have any relevance when it comes to changing your appearance? Yes, of course. If we want to appeal to people, we can tailor our looks to fit in with these scientifically proven markers of attractiveness. Many women with overly masculine features have discovered that, following surgery, they have found it much easier to find a partner (and now you can see why). People who, through no fault of their own, look angry or irritable (maybe because of furrows or hooded eyes) find they are treated more openly and in a more friendly manner when they have corrective surgery (and now you can understand that too). You can see too why someone who is ashamed of their teeth, and so doesn't smile widely and openly, is at a huge disadvantage.

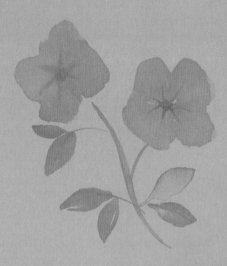

Change your appearance; change your life

It is obvious there is little we can do to change society. However we *can* change ourselves. So no wonder women are seeking the advantage that good looks can give. Many of the women who consult us find the glass ceiling disappears when they 'look the part' in the tough business world of the noughties. Other patients are over the moon because their new look has improved, or even saved, their relationship. Some tell us it has helped them find their perfect partner. It's one of those weird catch-22s: if you're happy, you attract more happiness to you like a magnet. If you're unhappy and gloomy, misery follows you like a stray dog. It also goes without saying that sex is bound to get better, *much* better, when you feel good about your body – there is nothing more sexy than someone who is happy in their skin, someone who has no inhibitions about the way they look. We cannot tell you how many times our patients have felt they have been given a second chance, a new beginning.

Bottom line: you *can* turn back the years.

You can change your face and body – and change your life. This isn't just based on anecdotal evidence. Solid scientific research shows that cosmetic surgery can improve your quality of life and your perception of well-being. For instance a study (reported in the *Annals of Plastic Surgery*) of patients following rhinoplasty (nose jobs) found that the majority of patients showed greater self-confidence and self-esteem in psychological tests following surgery.[*]

A further study presented to the American Society for Aesthetic Plastic Surgery (ASAPS), showed that cosmetic surgery produces a 'positive psychological effect, improving patients' quality of life and perceptions of wellbeing'. Not only did patients feel their quality of life was better but the study also showed that depression lowered significantly.[†]

This result was duplicated in a study in 2005 by the Aesthetic Surgery Education and Research Foundation (ASERF) which concluded that 'patients who invest their time and money in cosmetic procedures do experience lasting improvement in body image.'[‡]

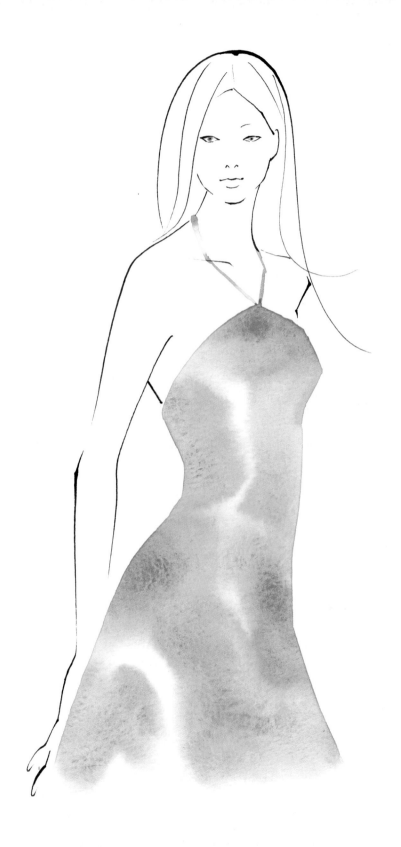

Using this book

This book is pretty different from other books on cosmetic surgery and anti-ageing. We won't be showing you gory pictures mid-operation because, frankly, who wants to see that? We will, however, be asking real people – just like you – to tell their stories, about what making changes did for them, how it felt, and whether it was worth it.

We would advise you to read this book right through, from start to finish. Having surgery is a big step and by working through this book you will be able to discover if it really is the right option for you, and whether you are thinking of the best possible procedure or procedures. We will be looking at the psychological reasons behind your desire for surgery, analysing why you want to change and which would be the best way to achieve the ideal end result. Don't be tempted to skip this part. You may think you know exactly what you want and why you want it but, from our experience, a lot of people change their minds after their first consultation with us. We won't be trying to put you off surgery, but we will be getting you to analyse exactly what you really need. We'll be asking you the kind of questions we ask all our patients here at the Centre – it's the next best thing to a private consultation. Quite apart from forming an essential part of your cosmetic surgery journey, it's also pretty entertaining and can be something of an eye-opener. You may discover things about your self and your life that you simply hadn't contemplated before.

We will also be very honest about what cosmetic surgery can – and can't – do. Yes, we have been told we work miracles – but some things are beyond the skill of even the most incredible surgeon. We have to work within the limits of the body and we can help you hone your expectations so they are realistic and achievable. We'll tell you the most common mistakes people make so you don't fall into the same traps. We'll also give you the honest low-down on the risks and side effects of cosmetic surgery; we believe everyone should go into a procedure with full knowledge of what it entails.

Most people think that cosmetic surgery is a lazy way to a perfect body or face. Certainly it can be a short cut to a better physique, but that doesn't mean you won't have to do any work. All reputable surgeons will ask you to get into the best possible health before you undergo surgery, which makes good clinical sense as it minimises the risks that automatically accompany any form of surgery. You may be asked to lose weight, to cut back on your alcohol intake and to stop smoking. At the Centre, we work closely with nutritional and fitness experts to ensure all our patients get the best advice on their pre- and post-operative fitness programmes. The other point about good diet and exercise is that they form the bedrock of rejuvenation. We can do a lot with the scalpel, with implants, fillers and peels, but you can help yourself a lot more by following our natural rejuvenation diet and finding your ideal exercise programme. The science of longevity is progressing in leaps and bounds: we'll tell you the latest research and how you can apply it practically in your daily life. We'll also be letting you in on the latest breakthroughs in anti-ageing medicine, particularly hormone therapy. Is it really youth in a bottle? Find out for yourself.

Before you commit yourself to any form of rejuvenation procedure or treatment, you need to be well prepared. We will advise you on how to get yourself into the best possible shape before surgery. We will also suggest how to find the perfect surgeon for your needs and tell you the absolutely essential questions you must ask before committing yourself. We will also give you guidelines on the optimum times to have each kind of surgery: why some procedures are better suited to fifty-somethings than thirty-somethings, why what works for a twenty-year-old might not be such a good choice for a woman in her forties.

Next we look at the burgeoning field of non-invasive procedures. It isn't always necessary to have full-blown invasive surgery – there are now a host of wonderful new procedures that give incredible effects with minimum trauma and side effects. Some people call these 'lunchtime fixes' as many of them barely disrupt your life. The problem is that there are now so many of these procedures, it can be tough to know where to start and which to trust. We will make it as simple and clear as possible.

Then we discuss major surgery. This is the definitive guide to the major forms of surgery. We have, over the years, learned exactly what every potential patient wants to know. So, we will tell you absolutely everything: how long the procedure takes, what kind of anaesthetic you will need, what your surgeon will do (without getting too gory) and whether you will need to stay in hospital (and if so, for how long). We will explain how long your recovery time will be, when you will see results, and we will warn you about any side effects and contraindications (when you shouldn't have a particular procedure). We will tell you whether you should expect stitches and scarring (and, if so, for how long); whether you will experience bruising, swelling and how much discomfort is involved. Really, we have thought of everything because these are the questions we answer each and every day in the course of our work.

The process of changing your face or body doesn't end when you leave the hospital or clinic. Many people find this post-operative stage of the process the hardest of all. Surgery has a psychological effect, as well as a physiological one. So you need to be prepared for how you will feel, inside, after you have shifted your exterior look. This is an exciting, yet also possibly frightening, time. Towards the end of the book, we'll help you adapt to your new look so you don't feel let down or alone. We'll also guide you through your healing process, advising on the best foods and supplements to take to let your body heal as swiftly and well as possible. We'll also provide you with your post-surgery life plan, a power programme that will help you keep yourself looking younger for longer. Finishing touches are important: we'll talk about make-up, hair, clothes and even posture to polish the new you.

Sounds good? Let's get started.

* *Annals of Plastic Surgery*, 27:3, 1991, September, 210–15.
† Study presented to the American Society for Aesthetic Plastic Surgery (ASAPS), 1997.
‡ *Aesthetic Surgery Journal (ASJ)*, 2005, May/June.

CHAPTER TWO

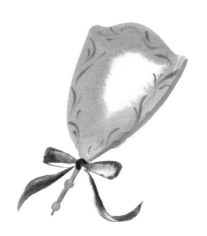

Why do you want
to change your looks?

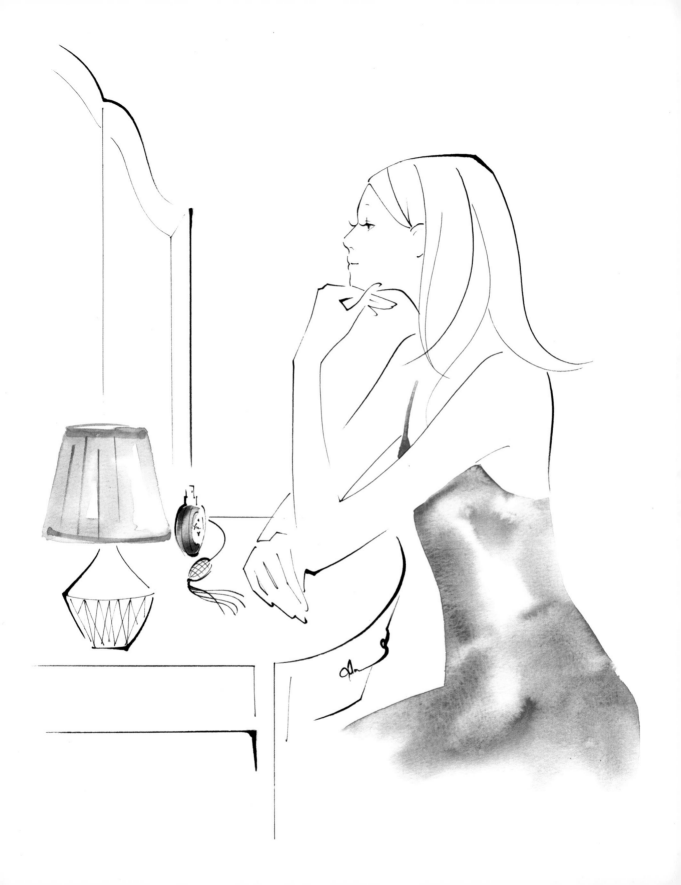

Everyone wants to look more beautiful. It's a given. But there are many ways of becoming more beautiful, and not all of them involve surgery. When someone comes into our clinic wanting cosmetic surgery, the first thing we do is talk. Then we talk some more. And then a bit more. In fact we often find we spend nearly as much time talking as we do operating. It's essential, a fundamental part of the process, because it is crucial to understand exactly why you want a procedure, what you expect from it, and how you think it will affect you. Any reputable surgeon will be just as keen on the talking bit as we are. If your prospective surgeon *doesn't* ask questions, if you *aren't* quizzed on your reasons for surgery, and your expectations, we would gently suggest you should look elsewhere. Not everyone is a suitable candidate for cosmetic surgery; in fact, as we'll explain, some people should actively avoid it. Some people have unrealistic expectations and can end up hugely disappointed or even angry about the results of their surgery – all of which could easily be avoided given adequate counselling. Some people don't even need cosmetic surgery to fulfil their dreams. Let's be honest, why spend more than you need, and put yourself through more discomfort than you need?

Our own stories

At this point, we would like to tell you our own stories, so you can see that there is no right or wrong answer, only the right answer for each individual person.

Maurizio: why I had surgery

I have had rhinoplasty (a nose job), botulinum injections (Botox) and fat injections.

I never liked my nose – it was simply out of proportion with the rest of my face and I wanted more harmony in my features. It had been bothering me for a long time and so, when I was thirty-one, I had it fixed (by Roberto of course!). Being a doctor, I wanted to experience the entire surgery so I decided not to have the usual general anaesthetic. It certainly was an experience, but not one I'd recommend to my patients – far better to wake up when it's all over.

As I got into my forties, I lost a lot of weight very swiftly and consequently lost a lot of fat on my face. It made me look tired and drawn all the time. So I had my own fat injected into my cheeks to make the skin look plumper and younger. It's a wonderful process, very natural and minimally invasive. Botulinum? Well, why have lines if you can get rid of them with one simple injection?

It all made me feel so much better about myself, I liked myself more. I started going to the gym, building up muscle, adjusting my posture. Now I don't dislike my body any more. I feel more comfortable with other people and I feel happy with myself. I feel pleasure when I go to the beach, when I undress in front of my girlfriend. I feel my body now reflects how I feel on the inside. I feel great!

Roberto: why I haven't had surgery

I haven't had surgery because I feel quite happy with what I have. I like my looks. I simply don't have any major issue that I feel needs to be corrected. Yes, I have a big nose, but so what? It doesn't matter to me and I don't feel any need to have it fixed.

But, at the same time, I am very aware that I have to preserve what I have; I have to work to delay the ageing process. Like everyone, I need some help. So I make sure my lifestyle is as good as it can possibly be. I work out at the gym and I have a really good diet. I drink lots of water and take care of my skin – I keep it hydrated and use great creams. I also make sure I keep happy as that is essential for looking and feeling young.

At the moment I am satisfied using totally natural ways to keep myself in good shape. However, I know the time will come when I'll need a bit more help and then, of course, I will do something about it.

Be prepared

Before you even book an appointment with a clinic, it's well worth spending some time thinking hard about how and why you want to change your appearance. You may come to realise that this isn't the right time, or that you haven't chosen quite the right procedure after all. Or that there is one you hadn't thought of that would be much better. Or that you could achieve the results you want without the need for surgery. On the other hand, it may confirm that you really would benefit – and will be great preparation for your initial meeting with your surgeon-to-be. We heave a huge sigh of relief when we meet patients who have thought this all through and are clear about their needs and hopes. It makes our job so much easier. Yes, we can often work wonders but we are not magicians. Equally, we are not mind-readers, and nor are any of our colleagues. We need you to work with us. We need feedback. We need you to give it all some serious thought and consideration. If we're going to make you the best you can be, we need to be a team – and you're an essential part of it.

In this chapter we're going to investigate exactly what you want to change about your appearance, and why. This is the backbone of what we do before we accept anyone for cosmetic surgery or rejuvenation therapy, and you'll find our colleagues (at least the good ones) all do the same. We want to be certain that you will get the most from your surgery, and ensure that we can give you the best advice on which surgery to have (or, in a few cases, when you really shouldn't opt for surgery). We would advise that, at this stage, you buy yourself a folder for all the information you will be gathering. You could use a ring binder or put loose sheets in a folder. A notebook would also be useful for the answers to your questions, and for jotting down any thoughts. This is also a place to note queries you will want to take to your chosen clinic. Don't hurry this process: take some serious time to think about these questions and work with the exercises. It's also worth talking to your partner or close family about some of the questions and getting their input too.

Where are you now?

Time to face facts. Time for a little bit of brutal reality. Take off all your make-up and all your clothes. First of all, stand in front of a full-length mirror and really look at yourself (yes, you *do* have to). Try, as far as possible, to be impartial. Imagine you were looking at someone else's body, that of your best friend perhaps. You'd be honest, wouldn't you, but you would also be kind. You'd try to find bits that were OK, rather than launch into a tirade of how fat and ugly she was. Think like Trinny and Susannah from *What Not to Wear* – they don't mince their words but they always find a good point. Now look at your body and face with that mindset. Start with an overview of your body. Then move in close to examine your face. Make sure you have plenty of good light – no use lurking in the shadows for this exercise, however tempting.

- What *are* the good bits? Everyone has something that's OK about their body. Yes, even you. What are your strengths? However hard, find one part of you that is OK. Now go one step further, and find a part that's gorgeous.

- Be honest and realistic about the bits that aren't so hot. Instead of saying, 'I'm fat,' give an honest appraisal of the situation; for example, 'I'm 12 pounds overweight,' or, 'I have a 35-inch waist.' Instead of, 'I'm ugly,' try, 'I have saggy bits under my chin and my lips are thin.'

- Work through your body and face in this way, building up a realistic, objective (as far as possible) scan of your problem areas.

Fill in the following charts to analyse precisely where your problems lie. Tick the boxes that apply.

YOUR FACE

PART OF FACE	LIKE	NEUTRAL	DISLIKE	COMMENTS
brow				
eyelids				
under eyes				
ears				
nose				
cheeks				
jawline				
mouth				
neck				
teeth				
skin tone				

YOUR BODY

PART OF BODY	LIKE	NEUTRAL	DISLIKE	COMMENTS
shoulders				
upper arms				
lower arms				
hands				
breasts				
back				
abdomen				
buttocks				
hips				
thighs				
knees				
calves				
ankles				
feet				
skin tone				

Don't be tempted to skim over this – it's a vital step in the process. We are all unhappy about certain parts of our bodies, but not all of us are quite ready to make changes. Be open to the possibility that there are some things you could change right now, and other things that might need to be put on the back burner, or even left exactly as they are for good. We're willing to bet there are plenty of issues that would respond to a few lifestyle changes. Be honest and highly analytical. Don't fall into the trap, at this stage, of thinking how you would fix the problems, just spend time getting them into perspective.

What do you really *really* want?

OK, you can put your clothes back on. Let's delve a little deeper now. Take out your notebook and start writing. Don't censor yourself – nobody needs read this but you. Notes are fine, so too are drawings. You might write a few lines, you might find you write pages upon pages. Give yourself permission to write whatever comes into your head, however mad or unrealistic it might seem.

- What would you change if you could? Again, be very precise, talk in terms of exact shifts, not vague generalities.

  - How far would you really want to go?
  - What would be your ideal figure? How would your face look in an ideal world?

- How would you feel if those parts of you were changed for ever? Imagine you have that perfect body or face …

  - What does it look like?
  - How would it feel to be that person? Spend some time imagining the impact that look would have on your life.
  - What would the advantages be? What would the disadvantages be?
  - Who would like it and who wouldn't?
  - How would people react differently to you? Would you like or dislike that difference?

Question yourself deeply. It's easy to think in general terms: I'd like to be thinner, I'd like bigger breasts, I'd like a facelift. But that won't really do the trick. Make your desires as specific as you possibly can. Just as you did in the last exercise, break down your wants so they become incredibly detailed.

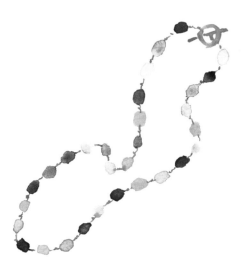

What does beauty mean to you?

Exactly what does beauty mean to you? Exactly what does thin mean to you? Reframe your answers so they are very specific. For example:

Old thought: I want to be thin.

New thought: I want to weigh x pounds, *or*, I want to lose 2 inches off my thighs, *or*, I want to get rid of the flabby bits of skin under my upper arms.

Old thought: I want to have a beautiful face.

New thought: I would prefer not to have large bags under my eyes. I would like to have fuller lips. I would like to have the bump on my nose removed.

Do you get the idea? Write everything down in your notebook. It's much more effective seeing it written down.

Remember that even the smallest changes will be very noticeable to you, because you are incredibly sensitised to your own body. Just how much is enough? Give it some serious thought and write down what you're thinking in your notebook.

Your surgeon can't choose your face or body

This process is critical as your surgeon needs to know what *you* need. All too often patients come into our consulting rooms and say, 'Tell me what I need, doctor.' No, no, no. *You* must decide what would make you feel better and more beautiful. You cannot abnegate responsibility. This is *your* body, this is *your* face. Of course we can advise you, we might even steer you towards better choices, but we cannot tell you what you should have. We don't expect you to know exactly which *procedure* would be best; it's our job to advise you on the best way to achieve the effect you want. But we won't decide what needs doing for you – only you know what you need to change.

It's also vital to bear in mind that rejuvenation is about making you look great – *you*, not someone else. If you would rather see someone else entirely in the mirror, we'd gently suggest you need to do some thoughtful inner work, maybe working with a psychotherapist to uncover why you feel such dislike for yourself. Cosmetic surgery is about bringing out the best in you. It's not about obliterating your old self entirely.

CASE STUDIES

Nicola Dixon, forty-two, is a natural health practitioner from Yorkshire.

I have been seeing the Viels for about five years now, and we have built up a wonderful relationship. It's very much like I have with my GP, my dentist or my hairdresser. I see them regularly and we discuss what needs to be done to keep me looking my best. I think there is a lot you can do with diet and exercise but, after that, if something bothers you, I'd say get rid of it. It's about inner respect.

I'm not neurotic but I do have a very artistic, and possibly critical, eye. My attitude is one of 'I don't like this about myself, what can we do about it?' I just go along and talk about it. But Maurizio and Roberto can be very strict and I have been talked out of procedures more times than I can remember. I thought I was looking saggy and needed a lift but Maurizio said, 'That's complete rubbish – there is nothing there to lift. You look fine. End of story. When you need a lift I'll tell you.'

There are plenty of surgeons who will do whatever you want, but you need to find someone who will get to know your skin, your psyche, your lifestyle and also think long-term. The Viels often won't do something because it would affect treatment I might need later. They like to keep things in reserve. So far, I've had liposuction, eyelid surgery, botulinum and fillers. I've had fat harvested and used to plump out my face. I also had a breast augmentation and went back twice to get my breasts bigger. The final time, they said simply, 'No, no bigger. You'd look like a porn star!' I had lost perspective but they could see what was going on, and while I think my husband was a little disappointed, I knew they were right. You have to trust your surgeon implicitly and be able to have an honest relationship. Frankly, they've got me for life.

Your cosmetic surgery, or someone else's?

We ask every one of our patients this very important question:

Do you want cosmetic surgery for you, yourself, or because someone else wants you to change?

Sadly, we see far too many women coming in wanting procedures because their partner likes bigger breasts, or fuller lips or whatever. Some women are even escorted in by their partners, explaining what they want. Some women, tragically, come along desperately wanting to shed a few years so they can compete with women ten years younger and hopefully prevent their partners from straying or 'trading them in for a newer model'.

Surgery is for you, and you alone. You need to feel 100 per cent happy with the procedure you choose and it must be *your* choice. So be honest: why do you truly want cosmetic surgery? What do you think it would do for your life? Complete these phrases (in as much detail as you can) in your notebook. Or get someone to ask you these questions or use a voice recorder – speaking can be more immediate than writing.

- If I had (insert your desire, e.g. bigger breasts/a smaller nose) I would feel…

- If I looked the way I want to look, I would go out and… … … … …

- If I had cosmetic surgery, my relationship would… … … … … … …

- If I didn't care what my partner thought, I would… … … … … … …

- If I could do anything in the world, I would… … … … … … … …

- If I didn't care how I looked, I would… … … … … … … … … …

Spend some time with this exercise as it can be very illuminating. Try not to censor yourself – just start the sentence and then write or say whatever pops into your head. It doesn't matter if it sounds silly or indulgent. We have found that people are frequently surprised when they try this, and some realise they don't really want cosmetic surgery. Others have discovered that they don't really want their partners any more! For others it just reinforces their feeling that a lot of things in their life would be more pleasant if they had a better self-image.

Your support structure

That's not to say that your partner or family aren't important. In fact, it's equally important to figure out the impact of your surgery on those around you.

- How does your partner feel about you looking younger/slimmer/different?

- How does he feel about cosmetic surgery?

- Are your family supportive of rejuvenation techniques and/or surgery?

- Have you talked about it with them?

Hopefully you will have strong support for any changes you want to make. This is very important for your post-surgery period, as the more support and help you have the swifter and easier your recovery will be.

If the people around you are not supportive, it is often through ignorance of modern rejuvenation techniques. They could be concerned that you will be in danger, that something could go wrong. Equally, they could think you will end up looking like someone else entirely, or that you'll have the dreaded wind tunnel effect or be a lookalike for one of the cosmetic surgery casualties you see in the papers. Reassure them. Let them read this book. Explain that this is something you need to do for your self-esteem and confidence. Give them the chance to express their concerns too; when they see the reality of modern subtle safe procedures, they'll probably change their minds (and may even book themselves in for a little nip and tuck). If one of the men in your life is very against cosmetic surgery (which can happen as men have had less exposure to information about procedures in the media), then point out to him that an ever growing percentage of our patients are men. Men too are realising that they can look so much better – and feel so much better about themselves.

Also bear in mind that change can be frightening for the people around you. Many partners with low self-esteem could be scared that a new more attractive you could be threatening. They might be scared that the power balance in your relationship could shift; they might be frightened that you would get more attention or even go off with someone else. Don't dismiss such thoughts: there could be some truth in them and these may be issues you need to think about yourself and work on together.

Why do you want to change?

Now we'd like you to look at your beliefs about beauty. As we've already discussed, we live in a society that is very driven by the way we look. Most of us grew up hearing statements about beauty and how people (particularly women) should look. It's worth investigating your own belief structure, and where it comes from. Many of us are still holding beliefs that belonged, originally, to our parents, our siblings, our teachers, even the editors of glossy magazines and film directors.

Think back to when you were a child.

- Which phrases or implied beliefs did you hear around you, concerning physical beauty? Can you remember? It could have been something like: 'Big breasts are womanly'; 'Only pretty girls are popular'; 'You won't get anywhere if you're fat.'

- Were you ever taunted about your face or body? Were you teased for having small or large breasts, or having your breasts develop early or late? Were you ribbed about your nose, or teeth? Were you given a hard time because you were overweight?

- Were you constantly compared to other members of the family? If so, was that a good thing or a bad thing? Did it set up expectations, or cause embarrassment? Some children even grow up feeling guilty that they share facial or bodily characteristics with a disliked family member. A common scenario nowadays is where a child of divorced parents grows up and inadvertently increasingly reminds one parent of the (disliked or even hated) other – you can imagine the psychological impact of that.

Write all these thoughts and memories down in your notebook. You may find this is quite an emotional process; children (and adults) can be very cruel and many of us carry hurts and sadnesses from childhood with us all our lives. Don't beat yourself up if you do feel sad. Feel empathy for that poor little child. It's incredibly easy to carry childhood belief systems right through our lives, but unfortunately it's not an effective way to live. Children don't always have the perception to make wise choices and it's quite possible you're struggling under outmoded, unnecessary and unhelpful beliefs. Time to challenge them. Look back at those beliefs with your adult hat on. How true are they? How valid and useful are they to you as an adult? Quiz yourself on what you – as a grown-up, not a child – believe. You need to be certain you are wanting change for your adult self, not out of a childhood need to please your playground peers!

CASE STUDY

Tabitha Cartwright, thirty-five, is a businesswoman from London.

I suppose I first became truly aware of the proportions of my nose when I was about twelve. I went to a traditional girls' grammar school and suffered a lot of unpleasant remarks. It was pretty grim really. I grew my hair long so it draped over my face and always covered my nose with my hand when I spoke. It was a huge drain on my self-esteem and confidence and stayed with me right through to adulthood.

Despite being very successful in my work, I didn't truly believe in myself, particularly when it came to relationships. I thought about rhinoplasty from time to time and I don't know why I didn't have it done earlier – partly I was too busy, partly I suppose I just didn't think I was worth it.

When my marriage failed, my self-esteem simply went into freefall. My husband had an affair and I just felt so unattractive and worthless. But then I realised I couldn't waste my whole life. It dawned on me that I had been a wife, not me. I never put myself first. So I sat down and wrote out a list of the things I wanted to do for me, just for me, and a nose job was top of the list. It was one thing I could control, one thing I could change, one thing I could do purely for myself.

It was quite an emotional journey. I didn't tell anyone I was having it done – it was something I needed to work through on my own. I also had some psychotherapy at the same time and my therapist was very encouraging and supportive: she felt it was a very positive step.

Maurizio spent ages with me, making sure I was doing it for the right reasons and working out exactly how my new nose would look. I wasn't remotely worried about the operation, I was just excited. I barely remember the operation or afterwards, but there were no real problems. I knew it would take quite a long time before my new nose would be its final shape but I was over the moon even when the dressing first came off.

It has truly changed how I feel about myself. I tie my hair back now and I'm far more confident. It's like I've shed something I've carried about for years. For so many years I felt I wasn't good enough. Now I know I am. I'm not going to live in someone else's shadow ever again.

The cult of perfection

What messages are we given by glossy magazines, television and film? Do you think those views are accurate? Are they valid? Our society praises and upholds beauty; it adores perfection. In this, it's no different from any other society – the only difference is that the concept of perfection changes from age to age and from place to place.

Think about what messages you are fed by the media. 'You can never be too rich or too thin' is the classic, swiftly followed by 'Youth is beauty'. Flick through any magazine and you'll have the message drummed in over and over: beauty equates to a long slim body, flat tummy, rounded firm breasts, young dewy skin, a pert nose and full sensual lips.

We're not saying you should necessarily turn your back on society's cult of perfection, but do see it for what it is. Recognise that the women you see in fashion magazines, presenting television programmes and acting in Hollywood movies just happen to embody the present-day cult of perfection.

What not to want

The one thing all cosmetic surgeons dread above all else is the woman who comes in, sits down and then merrily announces that she wants to look 'just like' Angelina Jolie, or Kate Moss or Naomi Campbell. Or that she wants Cameron Diaz's lips or Kylie's bottom and so on.

Why do we dread it? First because you can't just tack someone else's features on to your face. What looks great on one woman would look ghastly on another. Faces have proportions and if you lose proportion, you end up looking – to be frank – pretty odd.

Second, we want you to think about *your* face, *your* body, not those of a Hollywood celebrity or A-list model. Sure, we all look at the glossy magazines and appreciate the beauty of these people, but the best cosmetic surgery in the world won't turn you into them. Very *very* few women (maybe 5 per cent of the population) have the genetic luck to be born with what society now considers the ideal infrastructure. With the best will in the world, we will never be able to give you the endless legs of a six-foot model – no surgeon can. If you have a heavy bone structure, we can never transform you into a bird-like actress. We have had people asking if we could make their hands smaller (sadly impossible!); we get people who want their eyes a different colour (coloured contact lenses are your only option – we can't do it surgically); we even see people who ask us if we could give them a different shaped head (we can't). When you are assessing your body, please be realistic. Work with what you have, be smart about it and you can look great, whether you drew a long or short straw in the looks lottery.

It's worth remembering, too, that celebrities spend a small fortune in time and money on their appearance; after all, their faces and bodies are their livelihood. In reality, they work exceedingly hard to achieve that look. Most permanently diet (some nearly to the point of starvation); all of them have personal trainers and often work out for several hours a day to maintain their tone. Think about it:

How much time, effort and sheer hard work are you really prepared to give to your appearance?

Celebrities also don't always look as wonderful in the flesh as they do in the glossy magazines and on screen. We work with a lot of top models, actresses and television personalities; we see them without the make-up and in the flesh (rather than in touched-up photographs). We can assure you – and they would agree – that they aren't always perfect.

If you believe that by looking like your favourite celebrity you will magically attract their lifestyle, you're deluding yourself. It's tempting to think that if you looked like an A-lister you would automatically start to live that lifestyle, racing from party to première, from fabulous private yachts to front-row seats at fashion shows. Sadly it doesn't work like that.

So please, we beg you, make your desires realistic and based on you – not anybody else.

How would your life change if you had cosmetic surgery?

It's really helpful to think precisely what difference cosmetic surgery would make to your life. Why? Because it can help you figure out if your expectations would actually be met by having surgery, or whether you can meet your needs in other ways.

To ascertain this, we're using a highly effective technique from the form of psychotherapy known as Solution therapy or Brief therapy.

This exercise allows you to figure out exactly what you really need in your life. Give yourself plenty of time to do it. Sit down and ask yourself the following questions; or have someone else ask you.

1   Imagine you woke up one morning and found, to your amazement, that a miracle had happened and all your problems had disappeared overnight. How would you know the miracle had happened? Most people's first reaction is to say something like, 'I would look amazing,' or, 'I would be thin,' or, 'I'd have a wonderful relationship.' OK, but now try going beyond that and looking at how you would actually *feel*.

2   How exactly would you behave differently if a miracle had happened? You need to be as precise as possible. If you're still being woolly, keep going beyond.

For example:

– **Challenge: How would you know the miracle had happened?**
– **Response: I'd look amazing.**
– **Challenge: How would you behave if you looked amazing?**
– **Response: I'd have more confidence, more self-esteem.**
– **Challenge: How would you feel if you had more self-esteem and confidence?**
– **Response: I'd be more outgoing.**
– **Challenge: How would you know you were being more outgoing?**
– **Response: I'd talk to people at work. I'd start going to dance classes. I'd wear brighter clothes …**

Now these are actually all pretty good practical strategies – that you could do right now. Do you get the picture?

3   Now ask yourself how your family and friends would behave differently to you if the miracle had happened. Again, don't be woolly about this: how precisely would they behave, what precisely would they do?

4   How would *they* know a miracle had happened to you? How would *they* see the differences in your behaviour?

5   Are there parts of the miracle that are already happening in your life?

6   How have you got these things to happen? Could you get more of them to happen?

7   What elements of your life at present would you like to continue? What is good about your life? What works?

8   On a scale of nought to ten (where nought is the worst your life has been and ten is the day after the miracle) where are you now?

9   If you are on, say, four, how would you get to five? What would you be doing differently?

10 How would your family and friends know you had moved up one point?

The beauty of this technique is that it shows the ideals and dreams that lie behind our yearning for physical perfection. Most people come out with interesting results. They find that their deepest desire would be to have more loving relationships, to feel better about themselves, to laugh more, to have fun, to have more exciting sex or a more stimulating job. Others will be brutally honest and admit upfront that they want to wear gorgeous clothes, that they want admiration from other people, that they want more status and attention. Usually we find the bottom line is that most people crave an increased sense of confidence and self-worth, or simply want love or peace or security.

As we always say, changing your appearance can have a good effect on all these things, but you need to be aware that there are other ways of achieving the same goals.

This exercise will help you uncover how many of your goals for cosmetic surgery could be achieved without surgery, and, equally, what parts really do require radical action.

Bottom line: surgery or not?

By now you should have a pretty good idea if you really want and need invasive surgery, or if you are looking to improve your looks by non-surgical or non-invasive means. However, if you're still unsure, we have devised a very simple six-point questionnaire to determine if you're a good candidate for full-on surgery or not.

1   Are you over thirty? YES/NO

2   Can you afford it? Remember, it's not just the cost of the procedure you need to consider but also the cost of taking time off work/arranging childcare etc. YES/NO

3   Can you take the time off work? Can you manage on a day-to-day basis while you're recovering? Do you have adequate support? YES/NO

4   Do you feel OK about having surgery? Are you quite happy with the idea of incisions, anaesthetic and stitches? Can you cope with pain, discomfort and bruising? YES/NO

5   Are you in good general health, and not hugely overweight? YES/NO

6   Are you a non-smoker, or willing and able to quit? YES/NO

In order to be a good candidate for major surgery you really need to be able to answer YES to all these questions. Let's find out why:

● Research shows that the older you are, the more satisfied you will be with your surgery. There is increasing evidence that young people look on cosmetic surgery as a quick fix and expect that a refined feature or new breasts will somehow magically transform their lives. While some twenty-somethings do have very successful surgery (rhinoplasty and breast augmentation/reduction can be hugely life-enhancing for some young women), on the whole women in their thirties and above will be more content with their results.

● Cosmetic surgery is expensive and invasive procedures can cost roughly from two to ten thousand pounds. And you may need to add in additional costs such as any lost work time; childcare; taxis (following many invasive procedures you will not be able to drive or take public transport).

● It's essential to have a good support system if you're undergoing invasive procedures. You will feel quite poorly for up to several weeks following major surgery and will need help with lifting, carrying and everyday chores.

● It's easy to forget that much cosmetic surgery involves major intrusive surgery. You will be given painkillers but will still usually experience a degree (often quite a large degree) of pain and discomfort. You will be having yourself cut open and stitched up again. It's not for the overly squeamish.

- A good baseline of health can ensure your surgery carries the risk of far fewer complications or side effects. Many procedures will require you to lose excess weight before you undergo surgery; while we can remove excess pockets of stubborn fat, surgery is not a quick-fix alternative to a healthy diet and exercise plan.

- Smoking can cause you to heal far less quickly and well. We warn all our patients that if they smoke they will also run the risk of larger, more obvious scars.

If you feel uneasy about these points, don't despair. You can still change your looks, and your life, but in a slower, more holistic way.

The most common mistakes people make
In a nutshell, these are the most common mistakes we see, time and time again.

- Wanting to look like someone else: please, please, aim to look like yourself (only better), not some celebrity.

- Expecting miracles: there are limits, even with surgery. We can improve, we can delay ageing, but we cannot completely transform bodies and faces. Please get rid of unrealistic expectations.

- Going too far: a sign of good cosmetic surgery is that it isn't obvious. You should stay within the limits of nature – it isn't a circus. This applies equally to diet and exercise: you *can* be too thin; you *can* be too toned. Think harmony and proportion at all times.

- Losing proportion: it's far better to under-correct (then you can go back and do more) than over-correct.

- Expecting surgery automatically to change your life: you need to work on the inside as well as the outside.

- Wanting to lose too much fat: far too many women want to have every last inch of fat removed. They don't realise that if you remove all fat you age much quicker. Loss of fat is what gives you that tired look.

CHAPTER THREE

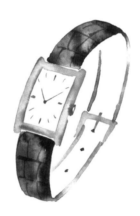

How and why your body ages

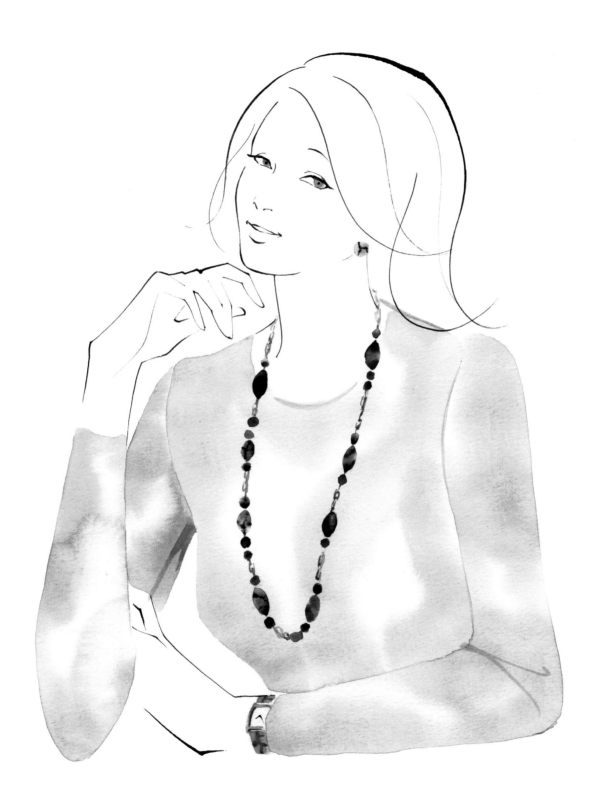

Before we look at precisely how to improve your looks, it's important to understand how ageing works. Don't worry, this won't be a long biology lesson, just the facts you need to know so what we talk about makes sense. Mostly this has to do with what happens as we get older. Obviously there are some aspects of your looks that have nothing to do with age. You might have been born with a very large or misshapen nose, for example, or you might have been unkindly gifted with tiny breasts, or overly generous thighs. In these cases, obviously, there is little that can be done other than specific surgery. However, the majority of our work is more a question of holding back the years and, in many cases, reversing them. The single most significant organ as far as the ageing process gives, is the skin, both on your face and your body.

What's your skin's structure?

Before we go any further, we need to explain briefly what your skin is all about. This is essential so that later on when we talk about the dermis or collagen or subcutaneous fat you will know what we're talking about. In a nutshell, your skin is rather like a slightly out-of-proportion wedding cake, with three distinct layers. Let's start from the top.

1   The epidermis. This is like the icing on a cake, it's the uppermost layer and can vary in thickness (it's at its thinnest on your eyelids, and at its thickest on the palms of your hands and the soles of your feet). It's actually subdivided into four layers (the stratum corneum at top, followed by the transitional layer, the suprabasal layer and the basal layer). Cells are produced in the lower levels of the epidermis and gradually travel upwards to the outer levels (on the surface of the skin) in a fifteen- to thirty-day cycle.

2   The dermis. Think of this as an exceedingly heavy-handed layer of marzipan under the icing of the epidermis. It's thicker than the epidermis and absolutely vital to how your skin ages. This is where your collagen and elastin live (in a ratio of 95 per cent collagen and 5 per cent elastin). About 70 per cent of the dermis is collagen, the rest being made up of elastin, blood vessels, sebaceous glands, hair follicles, sweat glands and immune system cells. The dermis also supplies water, nutrients and electrolytes to the epidermis above.

3   The subcutaneous layer. This is the cake part (although it's usually thinner than the dermis). It's made up mainly of fat, with blood vessels, nerve fibres and fibrous cells branching across it. Again, it varies according to which part of the body you find it in: for example your buttocks will usually have a pretty large subcutaneous layer while your hands won't. This layer helps maintain skin function. It's vital for youthful looks; when we start losing too much subcutaneous fat, we get hollow cheeks and scrawny hands. On the other hand it's the villain of the piece where cellulite is concerned.

Collagen and elastin

Protecting and promoting healthy abundant collagen and elastin are two of the major goals of beautification. But what are these wonder substances?

Collagen is a protein that forms the structural support of the dermis, creating a network of thin fibres. It plumps up the skin, giving it resilience, strength and the ability to stretch. It also helps to heal wounds and scars.

Elastin is another protein that weaves through the collagen to create a web of connective tissue, stretchy fibres vital for giving, as you might imagine from its name, elasticity. It also gives skin resilience and helps prevent it from sagging.

The cell factor

Each layer of your skin is made up of cells – good cells and bad cells, to put it simply. When we're young the fibroblast cells in our dermis make plenty of collagen, and also a small amount of an enzyme that breaks down collagen. Unfortunately, as we get older, our skin cells switch the percentages around, creating less collagen and more enzyme. The result is a disordering of the collagen leading to wrinkles and lines. As we age, our cells stop dividing and become 'senescent' (literally 'becoming older') and hang around causing damage to our skin.

One of the key factors in ageing cells is damage to the mitochondria (structures within the cells that transform the nutrients from the food we eat into a form that can be used by the body). This damage is caused by free radicals, created by oxygen reactions within the cells. The answer to free radicals lies with the white knights of the body – antioxidants. This is where diet becomes so vital. Powerful antioxidants can certainly block further free radical damage and research intimates that some of the new antioxidants being discovered may even be able to encourage cell repair and turn back the clock on damaged cells.

The latest research is looking into what actually triggers a cell to become senescent and the answer seems to lie in telomeres – the caps on the end of our chromosomes. Chromosomes are strands of DNA that carry the instruction manual for our cells, telling them what to do when. Each time a cell divides, a part of the telomere is lost. When all the telomere has gone, cell division stops and the cell becomes senescent. So, in theory, if we can stop the telomeres being eroded, we can stop cells ageing. This is the idea behind telomerase creams – add back telomerase and the cells will rejuvenate – although skin scientists are very doubtful that it could be delivered via a simple cream.

So, for now, we should be concentrating on what science knows works: a superb diet high in antioxidants; keeping our weight down (excess weight has been shown to decrease both health and lifespan) but not losing all of our essential fat; exercise to promote healthy circulation and hormone balance; and sensible supplementation. We also need to keep our stress levels down, and our sleep quota up – two more vital factors in the anti-ageing process.

The ageing process

It's a sad truth that as we get older our skin naturally and inexorably starts to sag and droop. Wrinkles, lines and furrows appear. Our skin may become blotchy, sallow, reddened or marked. It happens to everyone but what is interesting is that it happens at different rates. Some people age swifter than others. Why? Basically it depends on a clutch of factors. It will depend on your type of skin and your genetic blueprint. There is little you can do about those as none of us picks our parents! There is not a huge amount you can do about gravity either, which takes its inevitable downward path. However there are other factors over which you have much more control. It will depend on your exposure to environmental factors (predominantly the sun, but also pollution). It will depend on what you put into your body (food/drink/drugs/smoke from cigarettes). It can also depend on your mood. Yes, that's not a misprint – your emotions can and will affect your face.

The major causes of skin ageing are:

1   Sunlight

2   Smoking

3   Excess alcohol

4   Poor diet

5   Repetitive facial movements

6   Gravity

7   General ageing

8   Pollution

At first glance, this looks bad. But, when you look at it more closely, it's actually quite encouraging. Numbers one to four are all aspects of lifestyle that you could change right now. It's probably safe to say that only 10 per cent of your lines and wrinkles are unavoidable – the vast majority simply don't have to happen if you sort out your lifestyle.

Fine lines and wrinkles develop as the dermis thickens irregularly and also because of a decrease in moisture in the epidermis. This tends to be caused on the whole by exposure to sun and environmental toxins such as cigarette smoke. Don't believe it? Take a look at somewhere that doesn't get exposed to the sun and cigarettes – for example, your bottom. Any lines there? Any damage? Apart from the odd bit of cellulite (which we'll come on to later) it's highly unlikely you have a wrinkled, lined bottom. Do you take our point? This is, of course, a good reason for taking a preventative approach to skincare. However, don't panic: there is also plenty we can do to erase these lines, and stop them developing further.

In our business we talk about dynamic lines and static lines. Dynamic lines are the ones that appear when you move the muscles – for instance smile lines and forehead furrows. Static lines are those that remain the same without any muscle movement. Of course, given time, most dynamic lines will become static.

Your telltale face

It's fascinating that the type of person you are will show in your face. We can tell a lot about a patient's personality purely by reading the lines on her face.

- If you are a happy, easygoing person you will tend to develop crow's feet around the eyes (due to a lot of smiling and activity of the eyelid muscles, the orbicularis oculi).

- If you are an anxious person you will tend to develop worry lines on the forehead (due to contraction of the frontalis muscle).

- If you are an irritable or angry person, you will tend to develop frown lines between the eyebrows (due to contraction of the corrugator supercilii muscles and procerus muscles).

Please don't think we're advocating you avoid all expression. Our faces tell our history and give clues to our personality. When we look at a face, we don't think in terms of eradicating all personality, just enhancing the face's youthfulness. Lines aren't all bad. By the way, your face will also give away whether you smoke. You will tend to develop fine lines around your mouth, and crow's feet and wrinkles around the eyes. Not to mention a sallow, dull complexion.

What happens when

Every face is different. Every body is different. Everyone will age at a different rate, according to their genes, their lifestyle and their skin type. However, there are general changes that are more or less universal as we get older.

Time to take a look at what happens when in the lifetime of a face and body, and the lifestyle changes you can make that will help your skin.

Teens: the golden years. Skin should be firm, elastic and line- and wrinkle-free. Your dermis is lovely and plump, your collagen and elastin are being produced at an optimum rate and with maximum elasticity and resilience.

Trouble spots: literally, spots! If there's any blotch on your horizon it would be in the shape of acne, blackheads and whiteheads – the skin scourge of the teenage years. Blame it on your hormones which increase sebum. If you eat poorly and don't exercise you will carry excess weight, but this really shouldn't happen at your age.

What you should do: this is too young to consider surgery as your body isn't fully formed. However, your skin is never too young to be damaged. Take the opportunity to get into good habits (great diet, sensible exercise, optimum sleep) and don't be temped into bad habits (peer pressure may be tough to ignore when friends are smoking, drinking and eating junk food, but your skin will thank you later on for strength of character). Keep out of the sun or use adequate protection – sun damage can start in childhood. Make sure your skin is well hydrated and moisturised. Drink plenty of water and use a good moisturiser, one for young skin – it's not a case of the thicker the better – and you won't need intensive anti-wrinkle formulas.

Twenties: depressingly, skin starts to age from your late teens onwards. However, your twenties should see your skin looking smooth and clear. Fat should still be evenly distributed around your body although, if you do not watch your diet and exercise, your body fat will be increasing and muscle mass declining (along with a slowing of metabolism). Cell renewal starts to drop in your twenties and cells divide more slowly. You start to lose collagen at about 1.5 per cent a year after the age of twenty-five, as the dermis gradually becomes thinner. On the plus side, your hormones will have settled down and skin outbreaks should be a thing of the past.

Trouble spots: fair skin exposed to sunlight during childhood and teens may show sunspots and even early lines, in particular crow's feet.

What you should do: carry on with that diet and exercise plan to keep metabolism high. Don't fall into the trap of yo-yo dieting – it will wreck your skin. Your bones are still growing (right up until around the mid-twenties) so make sure you are getting enough calcium and the vital fatty acids. Keep an eye on your posture: long hours at a desk can wreak havoc (consider seeing an osteopath or taking Alexander Technique or Feldenkrais lessons: see pages 179). If you started smoking, quit. Start using a more powerful moisturiser. Exfoliate. Skin-brush to encourage lymphatic drainage (see page 64). Non-invasive treatments such as Endermologie, Beautytek, light peels and Lift 6 can give your skin a boost.

Thirties: everything you took for granted in your twenties is now a bonus if you can keep it. Keeping lean is an uphill battle as your body burns energy more slowly and your lean body mass decreases. Keep eating the same amount of calories and they'll head for your stomach and hips in the main. Skin becomes drier as oil glands become less active. The skin around your eyes starts to thin and collagen and elastin are breaking down, causing more fine lines and wrinkles to develop. Cellulite rears its bumpy head and fluid retention is more common. Some women find their hormones start to fluctuate. How you look in your thirties will depend very much on how much you have protected your skin from sunlight, and whether you smoke. Poor diet and excess alcohol will also start to show now.

Trouble spots: dull, sallow skin. Frown lines, crow's feet and other lines and wrinkles. Cellulite. Reddened skin and spider veins.

What you should do: keep up the good lifestyle plan and kick any bad habits (it's not too late). Consider non-invasive skin freshening techniques such as light peels and microdermabrasion. Botulinum at this stage will stop permanent folds forming from repetitive muscle activity (frowning, etc.). If you eat too much salt, cut it down – it will help with any fluid retention.

Check your sugar intake too as it can play havoc with your blood sugar levels and pile on the weight. Watch your alcohol intake – too much will bring on spider veins. Stress is often high in the thirties so make sure you have stress-busting strategies in place. Have your eyes tested: squinting can cause wrinkles. This can be a time for procedures such as LipoSelection, fat transplants and temporary fillers such as hyaluronic acid.

Forties: ageing starts in earnest now. Hormone levels start to fluctuate and many women will begin the run-up to menopause. Your skin is losing more collagen and elastin so more lines and wrinkles appear. It also loses subcutaneous fat, causing droopy baggy skin and making skin more fragile overall. Oil production lessens, making skin drier and more prone to wrinkles. You start to burn calories more slowly so, unless you cut back your calorie intake or exercise more stringently (or ideally both), you will put on weight. As you reach your late forties (and earlier in some women), your oestrogen levels fall, increasing the loss of collagen and elastin.

Trouble spots: weight gain (particularly around abdomen, hips and thighs). Less definition on jawline. Reddened skin and thread veins. Thinner lips. Nasolabial lines, frown lines and crow's feet.

What you should do: up your intake of antioxidants and ensure your diet is as good as it possibly can be. Look at your intake of oestrogen-balancing foods in particular. Exercise is vital to combat a slowing metabolism and maintain strong bones and muscles. Keep up the sunscreen and invest in more powerful anti-ageing creams and serums. Stress can be a problem in this decade, as can lack of sleep – take steps to sort out both. Botulinum, fillers and fat transfer can help restore a youthful face. Resurfacing (peels, laser, microdermabrasion) can be useful at this stage. You might also consider a thread lift or MACS lift.

Fifties: your skin is much more fragile and delicate now, due to falling oestrogen levels. Fat tissue continues to be lost, causing more sagging and drooping of skin, particularly on your face, neck and hands. However, in a cruel twist of fate, fat is more prone to develop around your waist, hips and thighs. Your bust size may also increase (breast size peaks from your mid-fifties to mid-sixties). Your skin will lose pigment and may become blotchy.

Trouble spots: lines may develop into folds. Eyelids and brows can droop, as can your entire lower face. Sunspots, blotches and dark shadows can become predominant. Previously toned areas (such as upper arms, thighs, abdomen) can become saggy and baggy.

What you should do: superb diet and exercise tailored to your individual needs is vital (try a personal trainer to get the best results). Increase flexibility with yoga or Pilates. Have your hormone levels checked and tailor diet and supplements to fix imbalances. Choose prescription-strength creams and serums that won't stretch your delicate skin. Resurfacing, fillers and implants are very helpful now and you may well consider surgery to fix serious sagging.

Sixties onwards: lines will continue to develop, depending on your exposure to sun and smoke. Sunspots, blotches and uneven tone and pigmentation may cause problems too. Weight will continue to be an issue, although you may notice you lose weight now from your breasts, leaving a sagging bustline. Skin continues to become thinner and more delicate, making it prone to bruising and damage.

Trouble spots: it can feel like your entire face and body become one large trouble spot!

What you should do: don't give up. Diet, tailor-made exercise and superb creams can do wonders. Maintenance resurfacing will keep your skin as good as possible (and looking many years younger). More radical surgery can give you back a firm face and body. Keep seeing your cosmetic surgeon who can advise on the best procedures.

THE LINE AND WRINKLE MAP

WHERE?	WHAT?	CAUSED BY
Forehead	Worry lines	Sun, frowning
Glabella (between eyebrows)	Frown lines	Sun, frowning, squinting, smoking
Eyebrows	Drooping brows	Sun, squinting, smoking, genetics, age
Around eyes	Crow's feet	Sun, smoking, squinting, smiling, dehydration, poor skincare
Cheeks, around nostrils	Reddening, thread veins	Sun, drinking, smoking, poor skincare, genetics, extremes of temperature
From nose to mouth (nasolabial)	Laughter lines	Sun, yo-yo dieting, sleeping on one side of the face, facial expressions.
Lower face, chin	Jowls	Crash dieting, yo-yo dieting, lack of exercise, hormonal changes
Around lips	Fine lines	Smoking

The five golden rules

Fortunately, there is plenty you can do to protect and improve your skin, whatever your age. If you do nothing else, follow these five golden rules. Not one of them involves any form of surgery. But they do require long-term commitment.

1   **Protect, protect, protect.** Use sunscreen, keep away from pollution as far as possible. Shun sunbeds.

2   **Keep away from smoke and alcohol.** If you smoke, quit. If you don't, keep yourself out of smoky atmospheres – passive smoking can age the skin too. Keep your alcohol intake low.

3   **Eat and drink your skin healthy.** Put into your body only foods and drinks that will help your skin, not hinder it. We'll discuss this in greater detail later on.

4   **Perfect your skincare routine.** Moisturisers improve the water-holding capacity of your skin, keeping moisture locked in. Gentle exfoliation can do wonders. It need not be complicated or expensive. Follow our simple plan later in the book for great results.

5   **Rejuvenate.** Many face creams and treatments now use wonder ingredients such as antioxidants, topical retinoids, polypeptides and alpha hydroxy acids to give your skin an anti-ageing power-boost. We'll look at these in more depth later.

A little extra help

It's easy to feel despondent, reading how skin ages. Don't be. If you follow all the golden rules, and still feel unhappy with the way you look, we have plenty of solutions to fix problem skin. These are the four major contenders.

1   **Resurface.** We can peel off the top layers of the epidermis using either mechanical methods or chemical peels, evening out skin texture and pigmentation. At the Centre we use chemical peels and dermabrasion. Other techniques include microdermabrasion, and laser resurfacing, including new techniques like the innovative Fraxel laser.

2   **Inject.** Botulinum toxin paralyses the muscles responsible for frown lines, crow's feet, smoker's lines around the mouth and forehead furrowing.

3   **Fill and implant.** A wide range of fillers or implants can fill deep lines, plump up thinning lips and fill out gaunt cheeks.

4   **Dig deep.** If the end result is still not satisfactory we can move on to surgical techniques such as facelifts, forehead, brow and neck lifts, rhinoplasty and blepharoplasty (eyelid surgery), which we'll discuss later in the book.

Your body blitz

As you age, your body loses its youthful, slim, toned look. Cellulite rears its ugly head too. We'll be looking at how to coax your body back to tip-top condition throughout this book but let's get the ball rolling by looking at the major factors that will keep your body looking young and feeling great.

1. Keep your weight down. **Nothing is more ageing and unappealing than excess fat. Research also shows that if you stay slim, you're more likely to stay healthy and live longer.**

2. Eat the foods your body loves. **Feed your body junk and you'll get a junk body. Nourish it with the best possible food and it will show a mile.**

3. Drink plenty of water. **A healthy body is a well-hydrated body. It will also help you keep your weight down – we often confuse thirst with hunger and eat when we really crave water. Plenty of water can prevent bloating and help you beat cellulite.**

4. Exercise – regularly. **No getting away from it: if you want a gorgeous body you need to work it. We'll show you ways to get yourself moving without pain, but with lots of gain.**

5. Keep out of the sun. **Just as your face will age in the sun, so will your body.**

6. Watch your posture. **Good posture can make you look slimmer and taller, can pull in a saggy stomach and can even improve your mood. No slumping allowed.**

7. Get fitted for the right bra. **Breast tissue is delicate and needs good support. The majority of women wear the wrong-sized bra and wreck their silhouette.**

8. Learn how to body-brush. **It will improve circulation, help slough off dead skin and, above all, boost your lymphatic system, helping to prevent cellulite and keeping your entire body in tip-top health.**

9. Detox from time to time. **Nobody's perfect and we don't expect you to follow all the rules all the time. But, maybe twice a year, give your body the chance to rest, recuperate and recharge.**

10. Pamper yourself. **Hydrotherapy, massage, aromatherapy, reflexology, body wraps and scrubs and treatments. They aren't miracle workers and don't expect them to do all the work for you, but they certainly can help (and, let's be honest, feel gorgeous too).**

Can you eliminate cellulite?

It's the question we're asked over and over again. Eighty per cent of women believe they have cellulite, so it's a big problem. While it's more obvious if you're overweight, even quite thin women can suffer, as absolutely every woman stores fat under her skin. Let's do some straight talking about the dreaded orange-peel skin.

Q: I've read reports that cellulite doesn't exist. So what is that on my thighs?

A: Yes, we've read those too but we've seen far too much cellulite to deny its existence. Cellulite most certainly does exist – without it, we'd have a vastly diminished practice!

Q: So, what is cellulite?

A: It's fat, basically, a type found deep in the skin that, very unfairly, targets women rather than men. It looks lumpy because of the uneven distribution of connective tissue around it. Some people believe that it is exacerbated by a build-up of toxins.

Q: So why do women get it and not men?

A: Some researchers believe it's a safety measure. The theory runs that cellulite is loaded with toxins and that if those toxins were easily released into a woman's bloodstream, they could compromise a pregnancy. So the stubbornness of cellulite protects a possible unborn foetus.

Q: I can't get rid of it with normal dieting or exercise – why?

A: You're not doing anything wrong, it's just that cellulite is very stubborn. If you follow the toxin theory, that will be reason enough for its tough stance. Others say it is a form of water retention – yet another reason why normal diet or exercise wouldn't shift it.

Q: So what can I do to get rid of it?

A: It depends on how much work you're willing to put in. You can tackle cellulite with a stringent regime of detox diet, exercise, skin-brushing and pummelling. If you're dedicated it should take about three or four months.

The other options are to use Endermologie or mesotherapy. Liposuction/LipoSelection does not remove cellulite although it can sometimes improve its appearance.

Q: I'm too lazy to do the long-haul option – what else is there?

A: Bioregenerative injections (mesotherapy) are minimally invasive (injections of hyaluronic acid and other active compounds are put into the skin to reduce the appearance of cellulite).

Q: There seem to be tons of beauty treatments that claim to treat cellulite. Do they work?

A: To be honest, it depends. Body wraps and creams generally only temporarily remove fluid retention, they don't seriously target cellulite. Treatments such as Ionithermie, which combine electrical stimulus with herbalised masks are very popular and can have good effects if combined with diet and exercise. Personally we like Endermologie, which uses mechanical means of zapping cellulite, and Beautytek, which uses advanced energywork. We use both with great results.

Q: I've heard that certain herbs can help cellulite – is that true?

A: Certainly a lot of anti-cellulite treatments and supplements contain herbs. Generally these act to prevent water retention, boost circulation and detoxify the body. The main anti-cellulite herbs include gotu kola, clover, bladderwrack, gingko biloba, dandelion and blue flag. Consider taking them in herbal teas – a good idea, as if you want to avoid cellulite you should also be avoiding tea, coffee and fizzy drinks.

CHAPTER FOUR

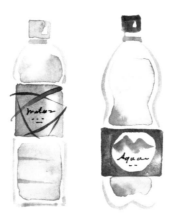

The Natural Rejuvenation Plan:
a new look without surgery

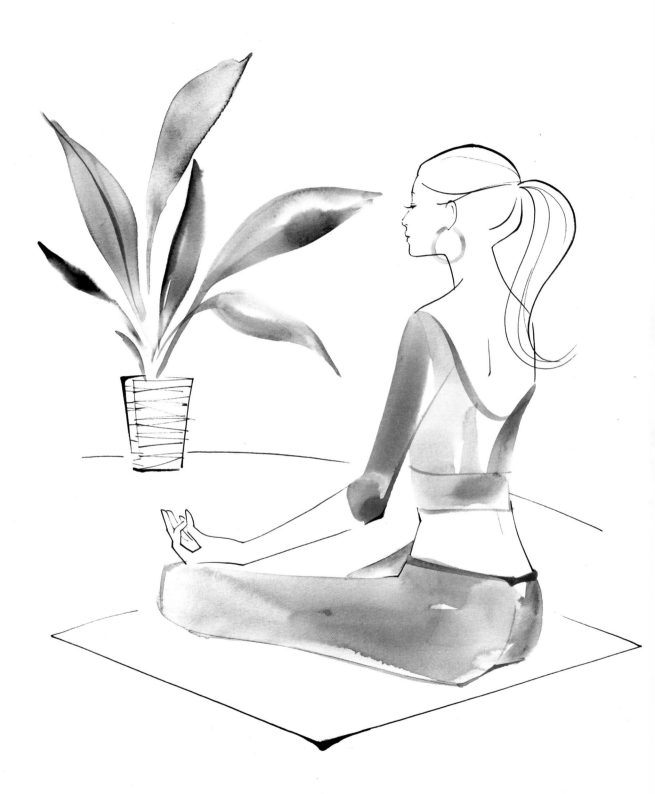

Allow us to let you into a secret. You don't always need surgery. Many people think the only way they will get the face and body they want is via a slew of invasive procedures. You can blame it on the extreme makeover shows which follow people undergoing a horde of procedures and emerging the other end looking totally unrecognisable. We all love a good transformation – there is something endlessly intriguing about seeing a stunning creature emerge from an ugly, or simply lacklustre, shell. It's a powerful myth: the clumsy caterpillar breaking out of the cocoon and transforming into the beautiful butterfly; the ugly duckling spreading his wings as a stunning swan. Physical change is startling and awe-inspiring, particularly when it happens overnight. Yet there's also something to be said for slower, more organic shifts.

Our Natural Rejuvenation Plan can make you not only look, but also feel, years younger. By working on diet, exercise, stress relief and your sleep, you can transform much more than just your looks: you can give your entire life, outlook and mood an overhaul. You will also give yourself a giant health boost, strengthening your immune system so you will be less likely to get colds and infections, encouraging your heart and lungs to protect you from cardiovascular disease, putting all your organs into tip-top working condition to protect you from a host of chronic forms of disease. You will automatically look good too. Our plan helps eliminate toxins from the body, it tackles free radicals head-on and helps promote cellular regeneration. Your skin will not only clear, but it will become more youthful. You will undoubtedly lose weight and will also crack the whip at cellulite. You will become not only more slender, but also more toned. This is no idle promise, we've seen it happen time and time again. Why should you be any different?

It may even be that, once you have sorted out diet and exercise, you might not need surgery after all. This one chapter alone could save you a fortune and might cut out (sorry for the pun) the need for any pain and discomfort. Then again, if you *do* decide you still want surgery, you will be in peak condition to gain most benefit. As surgeons, our hearts lift when we talk to a prospective patient who has done her homework and who is as fit and healthy as she can possibly be. It means we can concentrate on sorting out the bits that need fine-tuning, or which (with the best will and willpower in the world) simply won't respond to other means.

Your Six-Step Rejuvenation Plan

There are six essential components to our basic rejuvenation programme. They are, we promise, all incredibly simple and straightforward. There has been so much conflicting advice about what constitutes the perfect lifestyle but we will tell you exactly what to do and how to do it. Over the next few months we would like you to start transforming your life – and the way you look. It truly is very easy, this easy:

1   Banish bad habits. **Why you should ditch the cigarettes, shun the sun and cut back on alcohol.**

2   Eat well: the beauty eating plan. **We show you exactly what to eat – and what not to eat – to firm your body and clear your skin. Also which supplements you should take.**

3   Exercise regularly. **How to trim and tone yourself. Body sculpture without scalpels.**

4   Sleep your way to beauty. **They don't call it beauty sleep for nothing. How to get your best night's sleep ever.**

5   Seek serenity. **Stress ages us without a shadow of a doubt. Beat stress, cultivate calmness and you will shed years.**

6   Care for your skin. **Basic good cleansing and moisturising are the bedrock for good skincare. A few body basics too.**

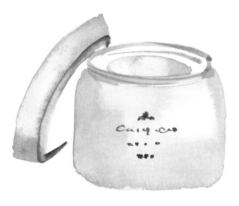

STEP ONE: BANISH BAD HABITS

Sorry, but if you want gorgeous skin, you will have to make a few sacrifices. We aren't killjoys and we don't believe in hair-shirts by any means, but we are quite adamant on a few distinct no-nos. If you want your skin to look its best, there are three things you should avoid: smoking, sun and excessive alcohol. So, before you do anything else, you need to lose those bad, skin-hurting habits. Sunlight and smoking are the two most damaging things you can do to your skin so it makes sense that you should knock those out before you even start looking at anything else. We're aware we're asking a lot – smoking is a huge addiction. But we would beg you to find a way of quitting. You can still follow the rest of the programme while continuing to smoke but sadly it just won't have the incredible effects it will have on non-smokers.

Unsophisticated Smoking

Can you smoke and be beautiful? Simple answer: no. Sorry. You might think you can get away with smoking when you are young (plenty of models and actresses act as role models there) but it will always tell on you in the end. A forty-year-old smoker can be as wrinkled as a sixty-year-old non-smoker. We're not being alarmist: it's a simple fact. Let's look at what smoking does to your skin:

- The chemicals in cigarettes trigger the release of those enzymes within the cells that reduce your skin's natural elasticity, breaking down collagen and consequently causing wrinkles, sagging and a sallow complexion. Research shows that smoking can reduce the production of collagen by up to 40 per cent, and once the collagen has gone, you'll need hard work to restimulate its growth. Yes, we have procedures that can help, but doesn't it make sense not to lose the collagen in the first place?

- Smoking leaches vitamins (in particular vitamins A and C) from the skin. These are two of the most potent anti-ageing vitamins, responsible for mopping up the free radicals that cause ageing and skin deterioration.

- Wrinkles and lines come about through repeated actions – hence the fact so many of us have frown lines. Think about what happens when you smoke. You purse your lips around your cigarette, sucking on it, so it should be no surprise that smokers tend to accumulate lines around the lips. Because smoke tends to get in your eyes, smokers squint a lot and – yes, you've got it – end up with awful crow's feet and that characteristic furrow between the eyebrows.

- The continual sucking when you draw on your cigarette will cause hollow, sunken cheeks given time.

- Smoking restricts your blood vessels, eventually reducing the flow of blood to the skin. Your skin becomes starved of oxygen and vital micronutrients and so starts to look sallow and swollen.

- The longer you smoke, the more your entire body suffers. Skin starts to look blue and bloated due to lack of oxygen and lung disease. Damage to your blood vessels can make your fingers and toes become white and aged. Eventually your nails will become deformed too. Of course, changes go on inside your body too: your heart becomes weakened, your lungs struggle to cope and you run a serious risk of heart disease, lung disease and cancer.

So, is smoking healthy? No. It's a recognised killer. Is it glamorous? Hardly. Is it really cool to suck on a bit of paper rolled around dried plant matter? Don't make us laugh. Do your skin and your body the best favour you possibly can, and give up. Yes, it can be hard. But studies show that high motivation makes giving up much easier. What is exciting is that you can undo much of the damage to your body and skin relatively quickly. The minute you pack up smoking, the damage to your collagen stops. Your circulation will also immediately start to improve and the levels of nicotine and carbon monoxide within your body will be halved just eight hours after stubbing out your last cigarette. You will see a clear improvement in your skin after only a fortnight and you'll be looking much better and feeling far more energetic after a month.

Use whatever it takes and whatever works for you.

- Your doctor can put you in touch with a local NHS group run by professionals trained to help you quit. This, combined with stop-smoking aids, can be very effective (making you up to four times more likely to stop than going it alone).

- Nicotine replacement therapy (NRT) in the form of skin patches, lozenges, tablets, gum or an inhaler can help. All give a slow release of nicotine to fight cravings.

- Zyban is a drug that suppresses the part of the brain that gives you the nicotine 'buzz' and doubles your chance of quitting. This is a prescription-only drug; ask your doctor if it might be suitable for you.

- Alternative approaches such as hypnotherapy and acupuncture can be very effective for many people.

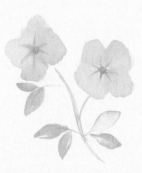

Your gorgeous super-ageing tan

Very few of us like the look of pale pasty skin. Who, in their right mind, wouldn't want to have golden sun-kissed skin? We are no exception. But, and we will let you into a secret, you will seldom find us lying on the beach or stretched out on a sunbed. If we do, we wear factor 30 suncream (and put factor 60 on the children). We're blessed with golden Italian skin and, if we need a top-up, we get it out of a tube.

Sunbathing is, sadly, one of the very worst things you can do to your skin. Sun exposure alters your skin genetically, leaving it wide open to ageing and even skin cancer. Along with smoking, tanning is the most ageing thing you can do to your skin, causing spider veins, brown spots, sagging, wrinkles, sallow skin and patchy pigmentation. It's safe to say that around 90 per cent of rejuvenation work is about trying to rectify the damage to the skin caused by persistent overexposure to sunlight.

UVA? UVB? Sorry, but neither is any good for your skin. Many tanning parlours claim their machines are safe because they use predominantly UVA light. While it's true that the UVB rays are the ones most likely to cause skin cancer, UVA isn't squeaky-clean by any means. UVA ages skin prematurely because it can penetrate down to the dermal layer where it breaks down both collagen and elastin, causing sagging and wrinkling. It can also damage the enzymes that protect against this breakdown. Add to that the fact that UVA light can also increase the risk of skin cancer, including the highly dangerous melanomas and I think you'd agree it's just not worth it.

So, what's the answer?

1 If you want a tan, fake it. No excuse nowadays – every salon offers tanning with no streaks and super-natural results. You're better off having it done professionally because home products (while much better than they were) can still leave you with brown knees and uneven patches. Don't be tempted by any variety of sunlamps, sunbeds or sunning kiosks, no matter how safe they claim to be. There simply is no such thing as a safe natural suntan.

2 Protect your skin at all times with a high-factor broad-spectrum sunscreen. Look for one that offers both UVA and UVB protection. UVA protection is usually indicated by a star rating, with four stars giving maximum protection. UVB protection is indicated by the SPF (sun protection factor) value; we recommend no lower than SPF15, and ideally SPF30. Apply sunscreen daily to all exposed parts of your skin. Waterproof is ideal, particularly for use on hands. While it may be tempting to rely on your moisturiser or foundation for skin protection (many now include sunscreens) we don't recommend that. To be totally safe, use a dedicated sunscreen under your make-up.

Awful ageing alcohol

Before you panic, we're not going to tell you to give up your Beaujolais or your Pinot Grigio – well, not entirely. All the research shows that a certain amount of alcohol (particularly red wine) has distinct health benefits, helping to keep your heart healthy and your stress levels low. Antioxidants called polyphenols, found in red wine, can really boost your health; in particular the antioxidant resveratrol is attracting a lot of attention. But, as with much in life, it's a case of a little of what you fancy, not a vat-ful. Push it too far and you'll be ageing your skin alongside your organs and the rest of your body. Guidelines suggest that you should drink no more than fourteen units of alcohol a week with at least one day a week being kept alcohol-free. A unit is a small glass of standard wine, half a pint of beer (standard bitter, not the strong stuff), or a pub measure (25ml) of spirits. However, if you want to lose weight, we'd suggest you give alcohol a complete miss – it really will pile on the pounds.

Heavy drinking is associated with accelerated ageing, with heart disease, stroke, liver and kidney damage and can be linked to breast cancer and osteoporosis. If that's not enough, the cosmetic effects are equally dire. Drinking too much takes its toll on your liver, fouling up its prime detoxification function. If your liver isn't working well, you can easily end up with puffy eyes, tired-looking skin, cracked lips, break-outs and acne flare-ups, plus dry lacklustre hair. Too much alcohol in your system also increases the production of free radicals while depleting your body of its complexion-boosting antioxidant micronutrients. To cap it all, alcohol causes enlargement of the blood vessels which, in time, will turn into reddening, thread or spider veins, giving that classic drinker's red face.

STEP TWO: THE BEAUTY EATING PLAN

Can food make you look and feel younger? Yes, absolutely. Every single thing you put in your mouth will be reflected in your skin. A sobering thought, isn't it? Diet really can help reverse ageing. It's a fact. It *is* totally possible to slow ageing and turn back the clock so you not only look more youthful, but your body actually *is* more youthful in real terms. When a patient walks into our consulting rooms we can always tell if she has a good diet or a lousy one. Your skin tells us all about your lifestyle and a diet packed with junk food, coffee and chocolate will stand out a mile. What is really exciting is that, if you do have a bad diet, you will be staggered at how swift and how extreme the improvement will be when you tidy up your act.

Do you need to lose weight?

The word 'diet' is synonymous with losing weight. It's also true that if you want to keep yourself as biologically young as possible, it's best to stay lean. Note, we say 'lean' not 'skinny' or 'thin'. Before everything else, you need to ascertain if you really do need to lose weight in the first place. Bear in mind that fat is never kind – it will never disappear from exactly the place you want it to, but will (perversely) cling there as if to taunt you. You may want to lose weight from your stomach or bottom but, ten to one, you will lose it from your face and breasts!

We would beg you not to become a super-waif. It's not attractive and is unkind to your skin and your body in general. Also, please believe us, it can be really ageing: fat loss is one of the first signs of ageing, producing sunken cheeks and a tired appearance. At the risk of sounding sexist we would also point out that most men don't find the waif a good look.

The best way to find out if you are overweight is to have your body fat measured, which can be done by using callipers. Our nutrition and exercise coach insists this is the only truly accurate way.

However the body mass index (BMI) will give you a rough idea and – unless you have a large amount of muscle – will be accurate enough.

All it takes is one simple equation (you might need a calculator or there are numerous websites that will do the calculation for you).

Your BMI = your weight (in kilos) divided by your height (in metres) squared.

So, if you weigh 68 kilos and are 1.8 metres tall, your calculation would look like this:

1.8 x 1.8 = 3.24 (your height squared)

68 divided by 3.24 = a BMI of 20.98

This is what your BMI means:

BMI 16–17.9 =   underweight
BMI 18–19.9 =   slightly underweight
BMI 20–24.9 =   normal weight
BMI 25–29.9 =   overweight
BMI 30–34.9 =   obesity (level 1)
BMI 35–39.9 =   obesity (level 2)
BMI over 40   =   extreme obesity (level 3)

It's all pretty self-explanatory. The ideal is a BMI of between 18 and 25. If your BMI lies within that bracket (and particularly if your BMI is below that threshold, making you underweight), you should not be seeking to spot-reduce by serious dieting. Exercise can help tone and trim problem areas or you may need cosmetic procedures to produce your ideal body. If, however, your BMI is over that level, you should think in terms of losing weight with diet and exercise before turning to cosmetic procedures. If you are clinically obese, we (and any other surgeon) would always expect you to lose weight before we would perform most cosmetic surgery.

How to lose weight: the 7-point simplicity plan

If you did need to lose weight, we would put you on a simple, effective weight-loss regime. We're loath to call it a diet as such, as everyone knows stringent diets simply don't work. This plan, however, does.

It's based around the principles of the Zone diet, made popular by Barry Sears, PhD. It is a very healthy regime and not remotely faddy. It simply adjusts the amounts of the foodstuffs we eat to promote weight loss. We would certainly recommend Barry Sears's books for more detailed information.

First and foremost you should take into account the GL (glycaemic load) of your diet. You're probably already aware of the concept of the GI (glycaemic index) of foods: basically how fast any individual carbohydrate-containing food causes blood sugar to rise. In a nutshell it teaches that we should be eating foods that cause our blood sugar levels to rise slowly and steadily (low GI, such as oats) rather than spiking furiously (high GI such as sugary cereal). Just when we'd got the hang of that, it became more confusing as researchers realised that many 'good' foods were (purely because of the way the load was being calculated) appearing on the 'bad' lists. The bottom line is that if you want to lose weight you need to keep an eye on the kind of food you are eating, and the amount of it you eat (GL). It's all common sense really.

There are seven simple points:

1   Drink at least 2 litres of water a day.

2   Drink two glasses of warm water twenty minutes before each meal to help with digestion, and to make you feel more full.

3   Have good quality organic protein at every meal (a portion no bigger and thicker than the palm of your hand).

4   Fill the other two-thirds of your plate with fresh, seasonal, organic vegetables.

5   Have a piece of fresh fruit with every meal – at the beginning not the end.

6   Add some cold-pressed organic oils for vital fatty acids – use as salad dressing or drizzle over vegetables.

7   Eat five small meals a day, making breakfast the biggest meal of the day.

That's it. How simple is that? Try it: it has worked time and time again with our patients, many of whom are desperate to lose weight (often because we won't operate on them until they do).

The Beauty Diet

If you don't need to lose weight (and after you have lost any weight necessary) we recommend you move on to our Beauty Diet. While our weight-loss plan is great and does its job, we do feel that you miss out on some vital rejuvenation nutrients by limiting your food choices quite so much. So, for full-on skin rejuvenation and masses of energy, we would suggest this plan. It's packed with the foods that your body, and in particular your skin, adores, and shuns all those that will age and damage your body and skin. Many of us eat a diet that will positively age our skin on a day-to-day basis. For example, the average person in Britain eats up to a staggering twenty teaspoons of sugar a day. It may taste nice but it's wrecking your skin, creating excessive free-radical formation which, in turn, plays havoc with your skin cells. Sugar builds up around the cells, where it weakens protein fibres, making skin weaker and more prone to sagging and wrinkles.

Let's start with what you *won't* be eating.

TEN TO AVOID

1   Sugar. Sugar creates inflammation in your cells, damages its collagen and also creates free radicals that cause skin damage. Check labels for hidden sugar (it lurks everywhere) and challenge your addiction to cakes, chocolate and sweets. You'll notice a huge difference in your skin.

2   Coffee (plus other drinks containing caffeine – tea, chocolate, colas and other soft drinks). Muddles up your metabolism, making it hard to lose weight and also contributing to ageing. Cut right down on alcohol too, especially if you are trying to lose weight.

3   'Bad' fat. Avoid all saturated fats (i.e. excess fat on meat), hydrogenated or trans fats (when oil is changed into solid fats, adding hydrogen atoms to the unsaturated fatty acids; they occur in most processed foods and many margarines) as they not only make you fat but cause change at a cellular level.

4   Additives. Chemicals are simply atrocious for your skin and your hormones, so shun all artificial sweeteners, preservatives, flavourings and so on. Yes, this will cut out most fast food, ready-meals and junk food. Avoid aspartame at all costs.

5   Fizzy drinks. Packed to the gills with sugar and/or artificial sweeteners, flavourings and other additives. Many also contain caffeine (see coffee).

6   Smoked meats, barbecued food. All loaded with hormones and chemicals. Also high in cholesterol and very fattening. Barbecued and burned food can also be carcinogenic (increasing your risk of cancer). Sadly, yes, this includes sausages, bacon, and all that lovely salami, Parma ham and coppa.

7   Excess dairy produce (butter, milk, cheese). A certain amount of dairy is fine, and it adds vital calcium and magnesium. However it is fattening, mucoid-forming and can cause congestion in the skin and organs. Some people are particularly intolerant of it. If you do have it, make sure it's organic.

8   Refined carbohydrates. White bread, white pasta, white rice. Empty calories on the whole and often stuffed full of additives. They also have a similar effect on the body as sugar.

9   Refined/processed salt. Atrocious for your blood pressure and causes water retention so you can expect bags under your eyes and generally puffy skin. Pies, pastries, processed foods, snacks all contain handfuls of it. Don't add it to your cooking or your food either. A little organic sea salt, however, is fine – add a pinch to your drinking water to fix the pH.

10 Processed or too much fruit juice. Surprised? Fruit juice can be incredibly fattening, causes energy spikes, and often doesn't contain the vital nutrients you think you're getting. You're better off eating the whole fruit.

TEN TO BOOST

Base your diet around these and you won't go far wrong.

1   Dark green vegetables. Natural powerhouses of antioxidants and other skin-loving and protecting phytonutrients. Broccoli et al. protect your bones, your skin and your eyes (as well as warding off cancer and heart disease).

2   All other vegetables and salads. The more (natural) colours you can get into your diet, the better. Think rainbow.

3   Super-fruits. Fresh organic fruit in season is your very best bet and packed with antioxidants and phytonutrients.

4   Organic protein. Fish, particularly oily fish, is great as it's rich in fatty acids (think wild salmon, mackerel, fresh tuna, sardines, herring and anchovies). Chicken, turkey and game are also good choices. Protein is vital in the good skin diet and if you don't have enough protein in your diet your skin will undoubtedly suffer. Protein boosts muscle tone and helps keep skin soft and wrinkle-free. It is essential for cellular repair. We cannot store protein in our bodies so ensure you have protein at every meal. It needn't come solely from animal sources – pulses, nuts and seeds are also good sources. You can also add two to three organic eggs per week.

5   Pulses, lentils, peas and beans. Packed with vitamins and micronutrients, they have wonderful anti-ageing properties.

6   Whole grains. Think brown and your skin will love you. A huge number of people are wheat-intolerant so think brown rice, spelt pasta, rye bread (also quinoa). Oats are fabulous too.

7   'Good' fats and oils. Not all fat is bad, far from it. Fats and oils provide essential antioxidant protection to cells. Cold-pressed olive oil and coconut oil are good for grilling or stir-frying food. Otherwise, use cold-pressed power oils such as walnut, almond and hemp in salads and added to cooked food to boost skin power.

8   Nuts and seeds. Natural, unsalted, these make a great antioxidant snack, and are another good protein source, but go easy if you're trying to lose weight as they are fattening. Make sure they're fresh too.

9   Dairy (in moderation). A little unpasteurised cheese is fine if you're not intolerant of cow's milk, but try out goat's and sheep's cheese as they are far more easily assimilated. Live bio-yoghurt teeming with 'good' bacteria can help clear your skin and enhance your immune system. Soya is very mucoid-forming so should be avoided and unfortunately rice and almond milk products are usually highly sweetened so none of these makes a good alternative.

10 Herbal teas and, in particular, green tea. These are packed with antioxidants and can help boost hormone levels too. Lemon or grapefruit squeezed in hot water is anti-parasitic and anti-fungal. Fresh mint leaves steeped in hot water are refreshing. Coffee substitutes like Barleycup, No-Caff and dandelion root are fine too.

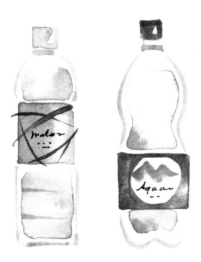

THE NATURAL REJUVENATION PLAN: A NEW LOOK WITHOUT SURGERY

If you're panicking about what to eat now we've taken away all those easy fast foods and comforting snacks, don't. Eating for optimum health and beauty is actually incredibly simple and fast. This is how you should be thinking:

- **Salads.** Throw together a huge bowl of salad stuff. Add protein (cooked and cooled pulses, lean meat, oily fish, etc.). Sprinkle on nuts and seeds. Toss in a little cold-pressed oil, flavoured with freshly chopped herbs. Easy.

- **Soups.** Chop up your choice of seasonal organic vegetables and throw into a pan along with herbs, spices and some protein. Cook, then blend (if you like a smooth texture) and serve.

- **Stir-fries.** Tiny dribble of olive oil in the wok, then toss together sticks of vegetables, strips of chicken or fish, sprouts (bean, pulse or seed). Add spices to give a flavour boost. Garnish with strips of omelette. Use coconut oil (anti-fungal).

- **Simply cooked protein.** Plonk your fish or meat under the grill or in the oven with a little olive oil to moisten. If you like, you can marinate it beforehand in olive oil with garlic and herbs. Serve with a salad or a pile of steamed or grilled vegetables. Poaching (in a little stock) is another great way to cook fish.

- **Steamed vegetables.** The less you cook your vegetables, the less vitamin C is lost (and the more your skin will like it). Vitamin C is your collagen's best friend so it makes sense.

- **Juiced vegetables.** Invest in a good quality juicer and experiment with different combinations. Juicing vegetables is the very best way to keep all their antioxidant properties. Wheatgrass and freshly sprouted grains, pulses and seeds pack a powerful health punch – add them to standard vegetables such as carrot, celery and beetroot. You can juice fresh fruit too but don't combine fruit and vegetables in the same juice. As with fresh fruit, juice should be drunk before, not after, meals.

- **Spelt pasta** with super-charged vegetable sauce and/or lean protein.

- **Paella, risotto, pilaf** using brown rice/millet/quinoa and whichever vegetables or protein take your fancy.

- **Natural live yoghurt** makes a great rejuvenation pudding. You can add a little honeycomb honey to sweeten.

- **Porridge** is a fabulous breakfast choice. Or soak organic finely milled oats overnight in milk and add nuts and seeds for a health-charged start to the day.

- **Vegetable-packed tortilla** is an unusual yet delicious choice. Or fill pancakes or dosas with vegetable, pulse or fish mixes.

We do not prescribe specific amounts of food on the Beauty Diet. Rigid diets, as we all know, simply don't work. We would much rather you learned to listen to your body's needs and re-educated your eating gradually. Everyone is different and so it's impossible to give one set of rules. However, these are guidelines that will suit everyone.

- Eat at regular times of the day.

- Don't skip meals, particularly not breakfast.

- Eat five small meals a day – build up gradually.

- Aim to include some protein in every meal.

- Make sure you eat vegetables or fruit at every meal.

- If you feel hungry between meals choose a healthy snack (some nuts or seeds are a good choice).

- Drink plenty of water throughout the day, but preferably not with meals. If you do drink with meals, choose warm rather than cold water.

- Eat slowly, chewing well.

- Concentrate on your food. Sit at a table to eat and don't be tempted to read or watch television (or any other activity) while eating.

- Stop eating when you feel full.

- Think about portion control. Your stomach is (or should be) about the size of your fist. Use a smaller plate so your meal doesn't look too meagre.

- Don't eat too late at night – certainly not after eight o'clock if you can help it – and keep that last meal small.

Eat this way, and with the foods we suggest, and you should notice huge improvements in your skin within a few weeks. If you need to lose weight, you will almost inevitably do this too, without any obvious effort. This happens because you will automatically be cutting out the foods that cause most people to put on excess weight. We follow the 80 per cent rule: eat really well 80 per cent of the time and don't worry too much if you slide once in a while. Just always try to keep in mind that everything, absolutely everything, you eat or drink will affect your health and the way you look.

WATER IS ESSENTIAL

We are watery beings – around 70 per cent of us is comprised of H_2O. Yet we're constantly amazed that our patients don't drink enough of the clear stuff. They're not the only ones: it's estimated that over 60 per cent of the population don't drink enough water for everyday health, let alone perfect skin. Think what happens to a plant if you don't water it – its leaves become thin and dry, and before long it starts to sag and droop. Without adequate hydration your skin will do exactly the same. Deprive your skin of water and you will, without a shadow of a doubt, look more wrinkled and lined as it loses its vital elasticity. Your cellulite, on the other hand, will plump up nicely without water! Even your hair is affected by your water intake, becoming lacklustre and dull if you don't drink enough.

How much is enough? Around 2 litres a day is the recommended amount. The best plan is to plonk a 2-litre bottle on your desk or kitchen table and sip throughout the day.

There is no real evidence to show that bottled water is any better than tap water (providing you use a good filter). In fact, water in plastic bottles could actually be bad for your health as chemicals and exo-oestrogens can leach into the water affecting, among other things, your hormone levels. So, if you do choose bottled water, make sure it comes in a glass bottle (and recycle it when you're done). The alternative is to install a reverse osmosis filtration system in your house, which is expensive, but does give you clean water.

REFINING THE BEAUTY DIET

We're asking you to make quite seismic changes to your diet. Take it slowly and those changes will become habits. Once you have noticed the benefits, you will most likely be so enthused that you will want to go a bit further.

So, for the real enthusiasts, here are a few refinements.

EAT AWAY WRINKLES

Antioxidants are your vital defence against ageing skin. All fruit and vegetables are high in antioxidants, but some are true super-foods. Oxygen Radical Absorbence Capacity (ORAC) measures the levels of antioxidants in a foodstuff. Here are the super-achievers:

Fruit	Vegetables
Blackberries	Alfalfa sprouts
Blueberries	Aubergine
Cherries	Beetroot
Grapefruit	Broccoli
Grapes (red)	Brussels sprouts
Kiwi fruit	Corn
Oranges	Kale
Plums	Onions
Prunes	Red peppers
Raisins	Spinach
Raspberries	
Strawberries	

Research shows that certain foods pack a hefty anti-ageing punch. Charge up your diet with these superstars:

1 Shiitake mushrooms (and other medicinal mushrooms, such as maitake, reishi, cordyceps). High in the glyconutrient n-acetylglucosamine, which can help balance hormones, regulate your immune system and even out oil production. Also contains mannose, which soothes inflammation in all cell membranes and promotes tissue regeneration. And fucose, which is vital for healthy cell structures in the skin. NOTE: button mushrooms have no health benefits.

2 Broccoli (and other green vegetables). Rejuvenation in a stalk. All green vegetables can help prevent cancer and heart disease; boost the immune system; protect bones and eyes. Contains galactose, which promotes wound healing and soothes inflammation. Also packed with vitamins and minerals including vital vitamin C, beta-carotene, calcium, folate and vitamin K. The phytonutrients sulforaphane and the indoles make broccoli special.

3 Aloe vera. Jam-packed full of active compounds including vitamins, amino acids and glyconutrients. Mix it with your own freshly squeezed fruit juice for a serious beauty boost.

4 Berries. All fruit is packed with antioxidants but fresh berries are real anti-ageing superstars, stacked with vitamins, minerals, phytonutrients and phyto-oestrogens. Blueberries are superstars. So too are pomegranates.

5 Beans (and pulses and peas). Chock-full of vitamins (particularly the B vitamins) and minerals, they also provide a fabulous low-fat protein source. They can help your heart, balance your blood pressure and cholesterol, and reduce your risk of diabetes. They are perfect diet food as they fill you up, keep energy levels high, but keep your weight down.

6 Oily fish. Packed with omega-3 oils, essential for preventing heart disease and cancer, while reducing blood pressure, easing arthritis and sharpening eyesight. Fatty acids also help preserve good skin tone.

7 Pumpkins (plus other squashes such as butternut, carrots, sweet potatoes). Full of carotenoids, super-antioxidants plus other vitamins and minerals.

8 Oats (and other whole grains). High in protein and fibre, vitamins and minerals, they can reduce your cholesterol levels and your risk of heart disease if you eat them regularly. They also balance out blood sugar levels, making it easier to lose weight. Oat bran is rich in ferulic acid, a newly discovered mega-antioxidant.

9 Almonds (and other nuts and seeds). Full of anti-ageing EFAs (essential fatty acids) and plant sterols (which can help lower cholesterol). They are also a great source of

antioxidants. Top nuts include almonds, walnuts, pistachios. Top seeds are pumpkin and sunflower seeds. Eat them as snacks, add to porridge and salads and use cold-pressed oil versions for salad dressings (but do not heat). NOTE: sprouted seeds and pulses are even more wonderful for your health.

10   Green tea. A powerhouse of antioxidants and flavenoids. Green tea really does seem able to do it all, from lowering your risk of killers such as cancer, heart disease and stroke through improving your gum and dental health, to boosting metabolism and helping you lose weight.

A FINAL THOUGHT: HYALURONIC ACID

We use hyaluronic acid a lot in our practice as a fabulous filler. It also crops up in plenty of cleansers, serums and moisturisers as a superb wrinkle-zapper and moisturiser. However it also occurs naturally in the skin where it helps keep moisture in the skin, and supports collagen and elastin. You can also boost it naturally by increasing your intake of the following:

- Beans/pulses
- Root vegetables such as carrots, parsnips, swede, turnip, sweet potatoes
- Stock made from chicken bones/skin etc.

Supplements

We firmly believe that supplements are a good idea if you want optimum health and beauty. However everyone's needs are different. At our Centre we work closely with a nutritional therapist and frequently refer our patients. We would strongly recommend you consult a well-qualified nutritional therapist so you can obtain a personalised plan. This is particularly important if you are planning to experiment with the new super-supplements we describe on the next page.

IMPORTANT NOTE: if you are taking any medication, have any medical condition or are pregnant, breastfeeding or trying to conceive you must always seek professional advice before taking *any* supplements.

THE SUPERB SIX

As a baseline you should think about supplementing the following:

1   A good quality multivitamin complex. Many are now packed with extras such as phytonutrients, blue-green algae, bioflavonoids and herbs. Look for supplements that use natural forms of nutrients (rather than synthetic substitutes). A good yardstick is that a decent multi will have a minimum of 25g of each of the B vitamins. Take in the morning.

2   A good quality multi-mineral complex. Look for one that uses absorbable forms of minerals (citrates, ascorbates or chelates) and contains at least 10mg of zinc and 30mcg of selenium. Take in the evening.

3   Extra vitamin C. Up to around 2g per day or to bowel tolerance (basically, if your bowel movements start to become loose you are taking too much so cut back).

4   A high-powered antioxidant complex. There are now many good formulations, generally containing beta-carotene and vitamins C and E; look out for those that also contain anthocyanidins, carotenoids, bioflavonoids, lycopene. The best will also contain many of the super-supplements listed below.

5   A good quality probiotic formula (beneficial bacteria). Ideally one that includes the prebiotic FOS, their ideal food base.

6   An EFA (essential fatty acid) supplement or oil to add to salads, soups etc. Ideally you should include the whole spectrum of omega-3, omega-6 and omega-9. Fish oils are good sources of omega-3 but don't be tempted to buy cheap supplements as they can contain toxic chemicals. Hemp seeds and flaxseed (linseed) are also good omega-3 sources. Evening primrose oil, borage oil and pumpkin oil are good sources of omega-6. You'll find omega-9 in extra virgin olive oil, avocado oil. Ideally, find a supplement that includes all three in balance.

There are many good brands of supplements available, including Biocare, Solgar, Living Fuel, Higher Nature and Viridian.

SUPER-SUPPLEMENTS FOR BEAUTY AND REJUVENATION

We all know that vitamins A, C and E are fantastic for your skin. But there are some new superstars in the rejuvenation game.

1   Alpha-lipoic acid: an incredibly powerful antioxidant that possesses a host of anti-ageing, beautifying effects. Because it is both fat and water soluble, it allows it to scavenge for free radicals in all tissues of the body. It helps to protect DNA and boost cellular energy. It also boosts the performance of other antioxidants. It can help prevent the breakdown of collagen and hold back wrinkles. It may also protect the eyes.

2   L-Glutathione: another super antioxidant, this amino acid is produced naturally in the liver. It is a staunch protector against the ravages of cigarette smoke, alcohol and other toxins. Levels decrease with age so a supplement is a wise idea.

3   CoQ10: a vital enzyme and antioxidant that lets the cell use oxygen in an efficient way by metabolising fats and carbohydrates. It has wonderful anti-ageing properties, helping to protect the heart, the brain and the nervous system. It also protects the skin. Our natural levels decline with age so it makes sense to supplement.

4   Acetyl-L-Carnitine (ALC): an amino acid that helps cells produce more energy, and also seems to protect against ageing. It can improve the tone and plumpness of your

skin. It is also vital for brain function, helping memory and acting as true 'brain food', boosting your thought processes. If that weren't enough, it also acts as a heart tonic and a general detoxifier.

5   N-Acetyl-L-Cysteine (NAC): a modified form of the amino acid cysteine, a powerful antioxidant that can help build connective tissue, detoxify the body, prevent muscle damage after exercise and reduce inflammation. It helps boost the immune system and generally combat ageing. It also helps to release, increase and preserve glutathione (see 2) levels.

6   MSM (methylsulfonylmethane): a form of sulphur that occurs naturally in the body. It is vital for healthy collagen production and also has profound antioxidant effects. Without proper levels of MSM our bodies simply cannot create healthy new cells. Sadly, unless we eat a predominantly raw food diet, we won't take in enough MSM so supplementation makes sense.

7   DMAE: a brain chemical that also acts as an antioxidant, protecting cell membranes. It helps to increase muscle tone all over the body and face, can improve skin tone and help prevent sagging and puffiness.

8   Grapeseed extract and pycnogenol: again, more powerful antioxidants. These also help repair connective tissue, strengthen collagen, improve skin tone, prevent wrinkles, strengthen capillaries and boost the immune system. They also have an anti-inflammatory effect.

9   SOD (Superoxide Dismutase): an enzyme that neutralises the superoxide radicals, the most dangerous free radicals in the body that break down synovial fluid and cartilage leading to inflammation and arthritis. Again, its natural levels decline with age and so supplementation is very useful.

10   Hyaluronic acid: hyaluronic acid is a natural component of skin, eyes and joints. Its aim in life is to bind water and lubricate the body and, in particular, the skin. Supplementing not only protects your joints but also gives a huge boost to the skin, making it softer and smoother. It also protects your eyes.

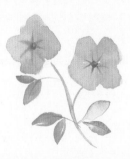

CASE STUDY

Kirsty Shaw is in her thirties and has a PR company. She lives in London and has three children.

Before I had my children I was always a size ten, and I weighed about 9 stone. When I was pregnant with the twins I went up to a gigantic 16 stone, and after I had my daughter I was still 2½ stone overweight. My whole body had changed, my skin was wrecked and I was desperate. I couldn't wear a bikini and I felt so depressed. No matter how hard I tried I just kept putting on weight. Having young children didn't exactly help my diet. When you're with children you're surrounded by food – basically a lot of white bread, white pasta and so on. Like billions of women I was eating with them and polishing off their leftovers. I had a solid diet of bread, flour, yeast and doughnuts!

I wanted a tummy tuck but Maurizio said he wouldn't consider it until I had lost the excess weight and so he put me on a sensible eating plan. It was basic food science, not crash dieting at all. I had to watch my glycaemic load, cut out simple carbohydrates and eat plenty of good quality protein and vegetables. I also drank tons of water. I learned how to listen to my body so I could tell when I was full. That was hard to begin with but once you've got it, you never overeat again. I was allowed the odd glass of wine or gin and tonic and, to be honest, it wasn't that tough at all.

In fact it was totally exhilarating as I lost over 2 stone in two and a half months. You know when you can't stop grinning? I was like that. It seemed like every time I saw my girlfriends I had lost another 6 pounds! I got back into my size ten jeans, and now even wear size eight. I lost the weight over a year ago and it hasn't come back. OK, sometimes I will go on a bender and eat a box of Crispy Cremes or overdo the vodka, but I quickly get myself back to balance. Basically I now enjoy food, and I can get on with enjoying my life.

STEP THREE: EXERCISE REGULARLY

Your fail-proof exercise plan

What's one of the major factors that makes us look old? Loss of muscle tone and mass. What builds muscle mass and tones muscles? Exercise, plus a good diet. Sorry, but it's the, possibly unpalatable, truth. We can give you a good shape with cosmetic surgery but if you want a truly great shape, you'll need to do a bit of work.

Regular exercise with sensible focused workouts can actually turn back the years. We aren't joking; after a year of regular sensible exercising, you can literally make your body up to twenty years younger. The magic combination of weight-training and cardiovascular (aerobic) exercise will boost your metabolism (making it easier to lose weight), build up bone density (so you aren't so likely to suffer from osteoporosis), increase flexibility and build your muscles. It can help normalise your blood pressure and balance your hormone levels. Exercise is a proven stress-beater (and you may be interested to know that stress hormones actually contribute to weight gain). Exercise helps to oxygenate the skin too, improving its colour and tone. Add to that the fact that exercise boosts the feelgood hormones, giving you a natural high, and can even perk up your sex life, and it really is a mystery why the gyms aren't packed. We haven't even mentioned the other plus points for exercise: it can make you lose weight and can give you a totally fabulous shape. Forget bulked-up superman muscles, a good exercise programme will create a long, lean, luscious shape.

If the carrot doesn't work, let's try the stick. If you *don't* exercise, you are running the risk of premature ageing and illness. Bodies need to work, they need to be stretched. If you live the life of a couch potato no amount of cosmetic surgery can make you healthy. Equally, you will be doing your face no favours. Lack of exercise ages skin, causing fat to accumulate on your chin and jowls, making your skin sallow and giving it a bloated appearance. You'll be holding the door wide open for cellulite too – poor circulation and a sluggish lymphatic system are natural sidekicks to a sedentary life.

Exercise does take work. We won't deny that. But it needn't be a bore or a chore. You just have to be smart and find a form of exercise that suits you and fits in with your lifestyle.

Equally you don't have to half kill yourself to get results. Yes, strenuous exercise will improve your aerobic capacity (how well your heart and lungs work) but light to moderate exercise will still have a good effect on that, and has been shown to be just as good, if not better, at lowering high blood pressure, reducing stress and helping you lose weight.

Cosmetic surgery cannot give you muscles but a good exercise plan can.

We frequently refer patients to our nutrition and exercise coach, Scott Bryant, who gets incredible results. We asked Scott to give his best advice for rejuvenating exercise.

How much exercise do I need?

Bottom line? You should look at doing at least thirty minutes of moderate-intensity exercise on at least four days a week (with days off in between). Yes, it sounds a lot but truly it will transform your shape, rejuvenate your body and balance your hormones.

If you're starting out, take it slow and easy. Get a check-up from your doctor. If you have health conditions you may need to exercise under supervision, or choose certain activities rather than others. But everyone can exercise. In some areas, GPs will actually 'prescribe' exercise and many health clubs and sports centres have specific groups for people with, for example, heart conditions or for the over-fifties.

If you possibly can, invest in the services of a good personal trainer or exercise coach. They will tailor a programme precisely for your body type and will find ways of squeezing exercise into even the busiest schedule.

The foolproof exercise plan for a slim, toned body

A lot of people put a huge amount of effort into exercise and yet see poor – if any – results. They become discouraged, think exercise doesn't work, and give up. It's a shame as really it is all very simple. If you want to look great and be incredibly healthy, you just have to follow a few essential points.

1   Have your posture and your musculo-skeletal structure checked out before you start any programme. Your exercise programme will need to be tailored to any structural imbalance you may have. This is really essential.

2   Learn how to engage and use your core muscles. Pilates is brilliant for teaching this. This is vital so that you don't strain or hurt yourself or give yourself back pain.

3   Use weights. Weight-training will not bulk you out – women don't possess enough testosterone to form huge muscles. But it will give you the body you've always dreamed of, and it will give your confidence and self-esteem a huge boost. A good weight programme will provide a cardio-respiratory effect too, as your heart rate will increase as you work at the optimum level. It's vital you keep progressing (increasing the weight you lift). You must, however, ensure you have superb technique (make sure you find a gym or trainer who can really show you precisely how to work).

4   Do high-intensity interval training. Most gyms will simply put you on aerobic machines (cycles, steppers, treadmills, rowers, etc.) and leave you there for hours. You may be burning calories, but you won't be burning fat as this kind of training does nothing for your metabolism. It's far better to do short sharp bursts of cardiovascular work. Work really hard for a minute, then ease off for a minute, then hard again, then easier again. When this gets easy, progress to two minutes on, two minutes off. If you are working well, you should not be able to chat.

5   Walk. Walking is superb exercise – it's wonderful for your body as it is what we were designed to do (unlike cycling, or endlessly stepping). Make sure your gait and posture remain good.

6   Make time for flexibility/stretching. Every workout should include some flexibility work in the form of stretching. It helps to prevent injury and also makes for lovely long lean muscles. Develop your suppleness and flexibility still further and deeper with yoga, Pilates, t'ai chi.

7   Qi gong is a fabulous exercise system that creates incredible inner strength and also gives mental poise and peace. Well worth investigating.

Exercise facts and fiction

Q: I want to lose weight. Shouldn't I just diet?

A: Absolutely not. If you want to lose weight the very best way is to combine sensible healthy eating with a solid exercise plan. You will get better results much more swiftly because by building muscle you will increase your metabolism and burn fat far more efficiently.

Q: I don't want huge bulging muscles, so I guess I shouldn't lift weights?

A: Women only have 1 per cent testosterone, so it's impossible to build huge bulky muscles by weight-lifting. Lifting weights is a great way to build strength, and boost your metabolism to burn more fat. It is also incredibly empowering and most women adore the strong lean look it gives.

Q: Is it true that fat turns to muscle when you exercise?

A: No. Fat and muscle are two completely different things. As you exercise, you will start to burn up fat (you will keep the same number of fat cells but there won't be so much fat in them so you will look and feel thinner). You will also increase the amount of muscle you have in your body. When you lose fat and gain muscle you get the impression of a slimmer, more toned body, but your fat cells are not turning into muscle.

Q: Is it really necessary to warm up before exercise?

A: Recent research indicates it's not as vital as we once thought. However, warming up does reduce the risk of injury, and eases your body into exercise. We'd still recommend you do a good five to ten minutes of warm-up before strenuous exercise.

Q: What about stretching? It's boring and surely a waste of time?

A: You should always stretch both before and after a workout. It prevents you becoming stiff and sore after exercise and also helps to unwind you after a strenuous workout.

Q: Surely more is better? Shouldn't I be exercising every day if I want the optimum benefits?

A: Your body needs time to repair and rest, particularly after strength work. Most athletes tend to stagger their workouts, so they will work on their lower body one day, and upper body the next, allowing the muscles time to repair and build. Stick to working out about four times a week with time off in between for the best results.

Tips for motivation

- With the best will in the world, few of us are strong-minded enough to exercise at home. You'd be much better off going to a gym or a class than dodging the sofa with a home DVD.

- Get an exercise 'buddy'. Having a partner makes you less likely to wimp out.

- Make exercise a date in your diary. If you block out appointment times for the gym, class or walking, you're more likely to keep faith.

- Get all your kit ready the night before and put your bag by the door or in your car so you can't forget it.

- Join a team. If you don't go, you're letting the whole side down.

- Pick your exercise time with care. Morning, lunchtime, or early afternoon are the best. It's much easier to make excuses to skip exercise after work.

- Find a gym, fitness centre or studio close to home or work. If you have to make a long detour to get there it's offputting.

- Make exercise fun. Meet friends at the gym or for a game of rounders in the park. Swim with your children, play squash with your partner.

- If you're a gadget person, get yourself some gizmos. Pedometers, sports tools that measure your speed, distance and calories burned, plus the trusty iPod can make workouts more fun.

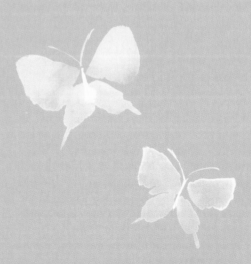

Seven ways to slot exercise into a frenetic life

So, you really don't have time to exercise? Try these:

1   Pretend lifts and escalators don't exist. Always take the stairs.

2   Take a brisk walk for ten minutes in your lunch-hour (or when you need a break).

3   Attack the housework with gusto. Vigorous hoovering, polishing, scrubbing and window-cleaning can be tough exercise. OK, few people will do non-stop floor-scrubbing for half an hour, but every bit helps.

4   Play games with your children. Chase, football, badminton, rough-housing.

5   Garden with intent. Mowing, sweeping, raking and digging all offer a great all-over body workout.

6   Fidget. Don't sit still if you can move. Pace around while taking calls or having meetings. Don't save your energy: jump up and down; walk over to see colleagues rather than phone or email.

7   If you can afford it, a personal trainer will find ways of seamlessly slotting exercise into even the craziest schedule. They will also be able to tailor a training regime for your individual needs and goals, and ensure you are always working at the optimum level. Truly, a wise investment.

Engage your core

This really is vital. Not only does it help give you a flatter-looking abdomen, it also protects your back from injury while exercising. It's incredibly simple:

1   Lie down on your back. Knees bent and hip-distance apart. Feet firmly on the ground.

2   Place your hands either side of your belly button, so your thumbs are touching your lower ribs.

3   Exhale fully and pull your navel back into your spine.

4   Feel every vertebra pressing into the carpet.

5   Now inhale. If your thumbs start to rise, your lower ribs are tipping up – exhale hard to re-engage your core.

After a little practice, this becomes second nature. Keeping your core engaged while exercising is a much more effective, not to mention safer, way of working out.

Exercise for specific areas of the body

It's nigh-on impossible to 'spot-reduce': if you lose fat you will tend to lose it from all over your body, or parts from which you are genetically wired to lose it. Tough, but true. However some strategies can help specific parts of the body.

FLAT STOMACH

Forget doing hundreds of crunches. You need to address your diet. These are the golden rules:

- Check with your doctor that you're not insulin-resistant.
- Cut out caffeine (tea/coffee/fizzy drinks).
- Cut out alcohol.
- Cut out wheat and dairy.
- Eat plenty of good quality organic protein.
- Get enough water.

When it comes to exercise, you need to build up your core muscles; use a Swiss ball for best results. These are three exercises to start you off:

Abdominal crunch on the Swiss ball

1 Put your tongue to the roof of your mouth, behind the front teeth, to stabilise your head, neck and jaw.

2 Rest the small of your back on the ball. Keep your knees bent at 90 degrees, and your feet firmly on the floor, hip-width apart.

3 Engage your core, pulling belly button to spine.

4 Slowly curl your sternum towards your pelvis – it's a small but focused movement.

5 As you come up, breathe out.

6 As you go back down, breathe in.

7 Repeat for about eight to twelve repetitions. Rest and repeat the whole cycle for two more sets.

Lower abdominals

1 Lie on the floor. Put your fingers under your back, rotate your pelvis and engage core.

2 Lift one leg up, at a 45-degree angle. Replace.

3 Then lift the other leg up, again at 45 degrees.

4 Continue, performing three sets of twelve repetitions.

Obliques (sides of the abdominals)

1 Get a dumb-bell (between 2 and 4 kilos, depending on your strength).

2 Stand with feet shoulder-width apart and engage core.

3 Allow the arm with the dumb-bell to slide down the leg on the same side.

4 Bring the arm back up (keeping the arm straight but not locked).

5 Repeat twelve times on one side, and then shift the dumb-bell to the other arm and repeat on that side.

6 You can carry out three sets of twelve repetitions.

FIRMER BUST
These exercises really can help to firm up the bustline, but they take dedication and hard work.

Press-up against the wall
1 Stand in front of a wall with your feet shoulder-width apart, about two paces back from the wall.

2 Place your hands flat against the wall, on a level with your shoulders.

3 Engage core. Push into the wall, and then back away from it.

4 Repeat eight to twelve times for three sets.

Once you have mastered this, and find it easy, progress to:

Two chair press-up
1 Place two chairs about 18 inches apart.

2 Put one leg on each chair, your hands on the floor in front of you and engage core.

3 Push up and down slowly with intent. Don't allow yourself to flop.

4 It's better to do just a few properly than loads with poor technique.

TONED ARMS
It is totally possible to get rid of the dreaded bats' wings with a series of dedicated arm-toning exercises. But expect hard work. You can use weights or resistance bands for these exercises. Start off small but as soon as an exercise gets easy, increase the weight or the pressure. You should always find it tough to do the last few reps.

Dips
1 Find a step or low table – about 2 feet high. Sit down with your back to it.

2 Now place the palms of your hands flat on the step behind you, fingers facing forwards, elbows bent.

3 Your feet are in front of you, about shoulder-width apart, knees bent. Engage core.

4 Press down on your palms so that your butt lifts up and you are supporting yourself on you arms and legs.

5 Now dip your body down so your butt nearly touches the floor.

6 Bring yourself up again, slowly and with intent.

7 Repeat eight to twelve times. You can do two further sets if you can.

Triceps kick-back
1 Stand, with feet hip-distance apart and knees soft. Engage core.

2 Bring your fists up to your armpits, elbows bent and behind you (a bit like chicken wings).

3 Now, leaving your elbows where they are, push your lower arms back and then return them into your armpit, slowly and with intent.

4 Repeat twelve times. Rest and then repeat for two more sets.

Biceps curl
1 Stand, with feet hip-distance apart and knees soft. Engage core.

2 Hold your arms straight out in front of your chest, palms upwards.

3 Make a fist around your weight or band.

4 Leaving your upper arms where they are, bring your fists in to your shoulders, slowly and with intent.

5 Return them to the outstretched position.

6 Repeat twelve times. Rest and then repeat for two more sets.

Fat-burning is essential for most large thighs. But these exercises can help build firm muscle to assist the process. Loads of women use step machines to firm the thighs and butt, but they don't really work. You need to work at squats and lunges with superb precise technique.

Floor squat

1 Stand with feet hip-distance apart, feet slightly turned out, knees slightly bent.

2 Place hands on hips and engage core.

3 Slowly bend knees into a squat, squeezing buttocks tight.

4 Slowly return to upright position, squeezing buttocks and tilting pelvis forwards (this is important).

5 Repeat twelve times. Rest, and then do two more sets.

Jump squat

This is a much more advanced move. Only move on to it once you find standard floor squats easy. It is incredibly effective at toning the thighs and buttocks.

1 Stand with feet slightly more than hip-width apart. Feet facing forwards.

2 Bend forwards into squat position, keeping your knees back behind your toes.

3 Touch fingertips to the ground swiftly and then throw up your arms and come up out of the squat into a jump.

4 Land softly with the whole foot.

5 Repeat for twelve repetitions – or work towards it.

You can also try walking squats: walk then squat, walk then squat.

Lunges effectively target the thighs but you need very good technique. Your core should always be engaged and you need to keep your feet in alignment with your hips, and your eyes looking straight ahead, not down. Ideally, learn this with a trainer.

The squats will also help your butt. But there are a few other exercises that will firm you up in the nether region.

Swiss ball leg lifts

1 Lie prone on the ball. Hands in press-up position. Engage core.

2 Lift one leg up slowly into a right-angle from your body. Hold for ten seconds and then slowly, with control, lower the leg.

3 Repeat with the other leg.

4 Continue alternating legs for twelve repetitions on each side. Rest, then do two more sets if you can.

Swiss ball glute squeeze

1 Lie prone on the ball. Hands in press-up position on the floor. Engage core.

2 Bring both legs up straight behind you, feet together.

3 Squeeze in your bottom and the backs of your thighs.

4 Keep core engaged throughout this and don't be tempted to use your abdominal muscles to help you lift.

The walking workout

The research is crystal clear: walking is quite simply a wonderful form of exercise. Performed correctly it can raise your heartbeat to around 50 per cent of its maximum which is good news for your cardiovascular system. It uses all the large muscles of the body in a repetitive manner allowing more oxygen and nutrients to get around the body. Brisk walking is, perhaps surprisingly, an effective calorie-burner. Stride up a 15 per cent incline at around 4.5 miles an hour and you will slough off around 500 calories an hour: a 7mph jog on flat ground will notch up just 439. You'll trim up as well: walking uses similar muscles to running (the quadriceps, hip flexors, calf muscles and gluteals) so your legs will soon become firm. However you won't run the risk of damaging joints and ligaments (as runners so often do). If you swing your arms smoothly and rhythmically you will also give your upper body a workout. And if you incorporate a few hills you can expect to really tone your thighs and buttocks. Put it all together and, if you walk briskly for just forty-five minutes four times a week you would automatically lose 10–15 pounds in a year without modifying your diet in any way. Here are the golden rules – they're so simple:

1   Start off gently with a manageable target and build up to a regular four times a week for a minimum of half an hour.

2   You need decent shoes. Look for performance fitness walking shoes; you need to be able to flex your foot to about 40–45 degrees.

3   Start by walking gently for the first five minutes. Then spend a few minutes gently stretching before stepping up the pace.

4   Walk in a centred fashion: imagine a straight line stretching from between your feet ahead of you down the road. Keep your legs parallel to this line and your toes pointing directly ahead.

5   Take the longest stride that is comfortable and let your arms swing naturally at the same speed. Make sure your shoulders are relaxed.

6   Breathe from your abdomen, not your chest. Inhale and exhale rhythmically and easily through the nose.

7   Don't go walking in built-up areas on days of bad air quality – you could do more harm than good.

8   Don't add weights to your walking workout as you could damage your shoulders.

Qi Gong: The Master Exercise

The Chinese have been using qi gong (pronounced chee goong) to soothe stress and build strength (both physical and mental) for thousands of years. Qi gong is not a martial art: it is a holistic system that combines breathing techniques with precise movements and mental concentration; its aim is total health and well-being – and an incredible energy boost.

Practise regularly and you could increase your energy levels, manage your stress and prevent or cure any number of chronic or acute diseases. You would improve your concentration and academic performance and gain increased creativity and inspiration. Your sex life would naturally perk up. Your weight would automatically adjust itself to the optimum for your body and your skin would become clear and healthy. For the icing on the cake, you could find yourself adding years to your life.

Qi gong works by cleansing the energy pathways of the body (the meridians) to achieve harmonious energy flow. Once your vital energy is flowing smoothly, almost anything becomes possible. It's rather like acupuncture without needles.

Qi gong is a precise discipline, demanding meticulous concentration and patience. It is also surprisingly tough on the muscles. Even if you regularly lift weights you will undoubtedly find your muscles aching after your first few sessions. And, while you won't burn calories particularly, you will find your body shape changes.

Qi gong classes are now springing up around the country and, if you can, it's really worth while trying out this extraordinary system.

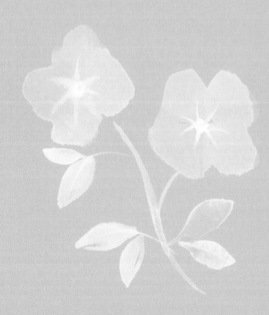

The Natural Rejuvenation Plan: a new look without surgery

CASE STUDY

Jemima Conway-Orr is thirty-seven and works as a designer. She lives in London.

I've always been very tall and as a child I had to have tablets to stop me growing too much. They left me a bit chubby and I've always had a layer of fat on my back. No matter how much I dieted I could never seem to lose weight from the right place. My face would start to look drawn and my arms would be skinny, but my back always looked immense – people thought I was a swimmer. Then, when I had my daughter fifteen months ago by Caesarean, I had a battle getting rid of that fat on my lower tummy.

Maurizio and Roberto recommended Scott Bryant, their personal trainer, and he really has done wonders.

To begin with it was pretty tough. But I soon started seeing results and when you start noticing fat disappearing and toned muscles coming in its place, that's a huge motivation. I see Scott three times a week (with a day off in between each session for the muscles to rest) and we do a variety of different kinds of exercise. Sometimes we do kick-boxing which I adore as it lets you get out all your aggression and it makes you really sweat. Or we might work with a Swiss ball, toning the deep abdominals. Then again, he might slot in some qi gong, for strength, focus and relaxation. The key is finding things you enjoy: if you get bored you simply won't stick to it.

I travel a lot for work and it's often tough to keep it all going. But Scott has shown me how to adapt our workouts so I can do them pretty well anywhere. You have to be able to incorporate exercise into your everyday life – it has to fit in or you simply won't keep it up. I think I have found a happy medium: my workouts are hard but good fun. Best of all, my shape has definitely changed. I have got rid of pretty much all the excess fat and now I look fit, but not bulky. My trousers are loose and I no longer feel bloated and uncomfortable.

I think exercise is vital, whether or not you opt for cosmetic surgery. It not only keeps you fit and in great shape, but improves your mental state, and is also a great insurance policy for later life. I'm hooked.

STEP FOUR: SLEEP YOUR WAY TO BEAUTY

They don't call it beauty sleep for nothing. If you want to look good and stay looking good, you need to make a regular good night's sleep a priority. While everyone varies to a degree, most people need about eight hours of good quality sleep. If you aren't getting enough, you will know all about it: you will feel tired, irritable and jaded, lacking in energy and unable to make good, clear, focused decisions. Lack of sleep can depress your immune system and also depress your mood. Your skin will show its displeasure with dark circles, puffiness and poor tone. Even your sex life may suffer: research has discovered that our sex hormones are suppressed when we deprive ourselves of sleep.

Remarkably little is known about the actual physiological effects of sleep but what is certain is that it drastically affects hormone function. In the first three hours of sleep large amounts of growth hormone are released into the body. Human growth hormone (HGH) is absolutely key in the fight against ageing. HGH basically keeps our bodies young – it coaxes the body to increase its ratio of lean muscle mass and decreases abdominal fat (the dreaded pot belly). It regenerates your skin, bones, heart, lungs, liver, kidneys, boosts your immune system and gives you a hefty dose of vital energy. It improves your lipid profile and helps prevent osteoporosis and arthritis. Truly, it's the elixir of youth; one of the Holy Grails of rejuvenation.

Ideally get to sleep before 10.30 p.m. because the sleep we get before midnight is the most restorative and rejuvenating.

As deep sleep ensues, more immune activities get under way. Other hormone levels rise too: such as prolactin, which is believed to regulate glucose and fatty acids in the blood, reduce water loss in the kidneys and generally balance our bodies. Melatonin, understood to influence regeneration and regulate water, rises, as do our sex hormones and DHEA, a steroid hormone, low levels of which are associated with ageing. On the other hand, sleep is the time when the stress hormones cortisol, adrenaline and noradrenaline decline (so lack of sleep means you never entirely switch off the stress response).

Appetite regulation is also linked to good sleep. Leptin, the hormone that tells us when we've had enough to eat, is increased while we sleep (and dramatically decreases when we suffer from sleep deprivation).

So, while we slumber, our bodies appear to be fine-tuning, balancing, protecting, above all *rejuvenating*. Lose sleep and you are losing one of your prime anti-ageing tools.

Top ten tips for a good night's sleep

Insomnia, the inability to sleep or sleeping poorly, is a modern epidemic. But if you want to look good, you need to sort it out as a priority.

1   Check there are no underlying psychological causes behind your insomnia (e.g. stress, anxiety, depression). If necessary, seek appropriate help (e.g. counselling, stress management).

2   Make sure your room is conducive to sleep. It needs to be cool and airy: stuffy overheated rooms can prevent sleep. Avoid having your computer or a television in your bedroom – it will distract you. If your room is very light (due to outside lighting) invest in blackout curtains as we need pure darkness for rejuvenating sleep. Earplugs can be helpful if your room is noisy. Make sure you have the right bed and, in particular, mattress. Mattresses don't last for ever – change yours at least every ten years. Make sure your mattress is neither too soft nor too hard. If you share your bed, have the largest bed you can fit into your bedroom (and afford) and you'll have less disturbance from your partner.

3   Avoid caffeine, alcohol and heavy meals late in the evening. Alcohol may send you to sleep but will often wake you up later or give you a disturbed night. Caffeine will stimulate the mind, and too much tea (or liquid in general) late at night will wake you up, needing to pee.

4   Ensure you are active enough during the day. We are designed to move around and a sedentary lifestyle can play havoc with your sleep. But don't go for vigorous exercise too close to bedtime.

5   Have a warm bath with essential oils. Use a few drops of oil mixed with a tablespoon of milk or sweet almond oil. Try lavender, Roman camomile and neroli to relieve anxiety and soothe. Bergamot helps insomnia linked to depression. Benzoin is useful when external worries are causing sleeplessness. These oils can also be used for massage (a few drops mixed with a carrier oil such as sweet almond); a gentle massage before sleep can help enormously.

6   Watch your diet. Low-calorie diets can affect the levels of your sleep hormones and going to bed hungry can cause low blood sugar levels, in turn triggering insomnia. Avoid refined carbohydrates, sugar, alcohol, tea and coffee, fizzy drinks and excess bran.

7   Try yoga, meditation and breathing techniques, particularly if stress is a factor. Progressive relaxation or visualisation can also help you relax (try the exercise on page 84).

8   Experiment with homeopathy. Ideally, consult a professional homeopath but you could also try the following (use the 30x potency available from chemists or health shops) if you suffer from these symptoms:

–   **Arsenicum Album**: feel sleepy during the day but wake at around 1–3 a.m. with anxiety or a racing mind. Restless in bed and often have anxiety dreams or nightmares.

–   **Lachesis**: menopausal sleep problems. Awful sense of the bed swaying or suffocation. Hold breath when falling asleep.

–   **Nux Vomica**: wake around 3–4 a.m. and not able to sleep again until just before the time you need to get up. Insomnia often caused by overwork. Drowsy in the evening.

–   **Pulsatilla**: wake very early with an overactive mind. Night sweats, feel alternately hot and cold in bed. Anxious or vivid dreams. Hate a stuffy room.

–   **Sepia**: have trouble falling asleep and wake up early feeling exhausted.

9   Try other alternatives. Acupuncture has a good record in helping insomnia. Hypnotherapy can reprogramme your mind into healthy sleep patterns. The Bach Flower Remedy, White Chestnut, can help if you can't sleep because recurrent thoughts whizz round your head. Herbs can help. Valerian, Passiflora, Rhodiola Rosea are natural tranquillisers.

10   If you are deficient in the hormone melatonin, you may find sleep a problem. You should consult a nutritional therapist or endocrinologist before supplementing melatonin (it isn't available over the counter in the UK anyhow). However you can boost melatonin levels by taking the supplement 5HTP, which converts to serotonin (a precursor of melatonin) in the body.

If none of these work, we would suggest you discuss the problem with your GP. It may be that a short course of sleeping tablets could help to break the pattern. Many varieties are now very mild and, if you take them for a short period only, won't be habit-forming.

How you sleep affects how you age

Ever thought your skin appears more wrinkled on one side of your face than on the other? You're not imagining it: most people gain uneven wrinkles because of the way they sleep. Look at your face directly after you wake up and you may well notice that you have lines on one side, particularly around the eyes. Generally these will plump out as the day goes on but, inevitably, as you get older they may become permanent. This happens because gravity pulls your skin, creating crumples on the side you favour. You can avoid skin wrinkles by lying on your back. If that's not an option, switch your pillowcases to silk or satin as these will minimise wrinkles (and they feel gorgeous too).

STEP FIVE: SEEK SERENITY

Stress statistics make for frightening reading: 75 per cent of the population experience at least 'some stress' every two weeks and anti-stress medication accounts for a quarter of all prescriptions. It's important to realise that not all stress is bad, and that a certain amount of stress is necessary for your adrenal glands to function properly. However, nowadays we tend to experience excessive, damaging stress, which results in an inability to turn off the stress response, leaving stress hormone levels (in particular cortisol) alarmingly high. The clinical manifestations of elevated cortisol are frightening: hypertension (high blood pressure); hyperglycaemia (which can lead to diabetes); bone loss; impaired immune function; muscle wasting; thinning skin; excess abdominal fat; water retention and bloating.

So, damaging stress can wreck your health and it will certainly play havoc with your looks. Let's be quite clear here: stress ages faces and puts strain (and weight) on bodies. It's been proven that skin actually ages faster during periods of emotional stress – a sobering thought.

In our frenetic modern world you simply can't avoid stress, but you can take steps to ensure it doesn't rule, or ruin, your life. We could write an entire book on how to keep your stress under control, but there is only space for a few pointers.

First of all, ask yourself a few tough questions:

- Are you doing too much? Analyse where your stress comes from and how much of it is truly necessary.

- What in your life could you delegate or share? Many of us hold on to too much as we are scared of letting go. Are you a control freak or a perfectionist? Maybe it's time to drop some commitments.

- On the other hand, do you have *too little* control in certain areas of your life? Stress comes from situations over which we have little or no control; a worker in a call centre actually suffers more damaging stress than an A&E surgeon for this very reason. Work out where you suffer from loss of control and see if you can claw it back.

- Do you say 'Yes' when you really want to say 'No'? Are you a people-pleaser who takes on too much because you don't like to let people down? Maybe it's time to put yourself first for once.

- Are you permanently 'on call'? We live in a 24/7 society but you can choose when and how you are contacted. Start turning off your mobile and turning on voicemail (answer in your own good time). Leave your laptop at work and keep clear boundaries between home and work. It's tough but vital.

Learn to relax

Relaxation is an art – and a vital one to learn if you want to look and feel serene. Learn this progressive relaxation technique to help you kick stress out of your life.

- Lie down, preferably on a blanket on the floor. Make sure you're warm and not in a draught. Start by becoming aware of your body, notice where it touches the ground. Notice anywhere you might be holding tension.

- Now tense your toes as tightly as you possibly can. Count slowly to three. Move on to your calves – tense and hold. Now you progressively move up through your body, gradually tensing every major muscle group in your body. Tense your thighs, your buttocks. Pull in your stomach and tense your abdomen. Make a fist and tense your arms. Shrug your shoulders. Screw up your face.

- Now take a deep breath in, hold, hold, hold – and let go.

- Repeat again, tensing right the way through your body, holding to the count of three and then let go.

- Now concentrate on relaxing your body. Wiggle your toes, let your feet fall apart. Relax your calves, your thighs, your hips and buttocks (check those buttocks really are relaxed – we hold a lot of tension there). Let go of your stomach, your abdomen, release your chest. Wiggle your fingers, relax your arms and let your hands fall loosely away from your body.

- Let your head gently stretch over to the right, then very slowly to the left, then back to the middle. Press your head gently into the ground to release the pressure from your neck.

- Now bring your attention to your face. Release your jaw (another prime tension site). Let the lines fall away from your face as it relaxes and softens. Imagine all the tension washing out of your face.

- Remain like this as long as you like, breathing deeply and evenly (but without strain). Let the breath gradually extend deeper and deeper, down from your chest into your abdomen. Breathe out all the tension; breathe in vitality, ease and relaxation.

- When you are ready, slowly turn over on to one side. Open your eyes and, in your own time, slowly sit up.

Ten instant stressbusters

Don't give the excuse that you don't have time to beat your stress! These stressbusters can be squeezed into even the busiest day.

1   Squeeze a 'stress ball', hand-sized squashy rubber balls available from health or beauty shops. The simple mechanical action of squeezing dampens stress and also massages hordes of acupressure points in the hand. Psychologists also found that popping bubble wrap can help reduce stress.

2   Use visualisation. Imagine yourself lying on a beach, listening to the waves, feeling the warm sun on your back (or choose any other pleasant place). Begin by practising at a quiet time when you aren't stressed and keep it up until you really know your place. Then, having set up your private refuge, you can escape into it whenever the stress levels start to rise.

3   Laugh. It relaxes your muscles and lowers blood pressure. It reduces stress hormone levels and increases levels of feelgood brain chemicals.

4   Put your elbows on your desk and put your face in your hands, cupping your palms over your eyes so your face is gently supported. Relax your shoulders and sink into the darkness for a few moments. Even just ten seconds can help.

5   When you've had a tiring day, spend a few minutes in this soothing yoga posture. Kneel down on the floor, with your knees together and your ankles relaxed so the heels fall apart. Allow your upper body to fall forwards on to the floor with your face on the floor and your arms loosely by your sides. Relax totally.

6   Mineral baths, such as Moor mud or Dead Sea salts, can help induce deep relaxation. Simply relax in the bath for twenty minutes then wrap yourself in towels.

7   Sit down, close your eyes and think of the person or situation that is making you feel stressed. Now imagine a room full of tables and shelves stacked high with plates, china, glass statues and the like. Go round and smash everything to pieces: hurl glasses against the wall; throw the tables around. Only finish when you have wrecked the entire room. You should feel a sense of relief after this exercise.

8   Exercise hard and tough. A really good aerobic workout allows the body's stress hormones to go into 'flight or fight' mode and then return naturally to their relaxed state. If you want to try something really challenging go for kick-boxing or 'power' yoga.

9 Delegate. You're not superhuman and you're not indispensable (however much you may like to think so!). So don't try to do everything. Stop thinking in terms of 'should', 'ought' and 'must' – if you choose to do something or want to do it that's fine – just remember you have a choice.

10 Bach Flower Remedies can help heal stress personalities. Try Impatiens if you're always in a hurry; Beech if you're intolerant and have to be right all the time; Vervain if you're a bit fanatical and over-enthusiastic; Olive for complete exhaustion and stress 'burn-out'. Available from chemists; follow the instructions on the bottle.

Anti-stress therapies

- If stress is a serious factor in your life, it's worth seeking help from a psychotherapist or counsellor. This needn't be a long-term, in-depth commitment: short, sharp-fix therapies like CBT, NLP and Solution-Focussed Therapy can get results fast. Your GP may be able to refer you.

- As emotional stress can cause ageing, it's worth getting your relationships on track. Couples counselling may help.

- Bodywork can release deeply held stress. Often our bodies hold on to stress long after our minds think they've released it. Look at osteopathy or chiropractic for body realignment. Rolfing or Hellerwork work on the fascia (connective tissue). Shiatsu and Thai massage release stress through deep stretching. Bottom line: any form of massage or bodywork will soothe stressed minds and bodies.

- Yoga and Pilates both stretch out tense muscles and are great stressbusters. Yoga often includes other stress-beating strategies such as meditation, deep relaxation and chanting.

- Floatation therapy (in a floatation tank) relaxes both body and mind, and is also said to increase concentration and creativity. Don't panic, it really isn't claustrophobic.

STEP SIX: YOUR BASIC SKINCARE REGIME

As you've seen, beauty really does come from within. What you eat, how you exercise, how you sleep and how you deal with stress are crucial. However, we'd be lying if we didn't tell you that you need to work on the outside too. Later on we will also be looking at the huge array of creams and serums on offer that promise serous anti-ageing benefits. For now, though, let's get the basics under control. We have some very good news. You really don't need tons of products, nor do you need to spend hours each day on your beauty regime. It's simply not necessary and all you're doing is adding to the coffers of the big cosmetic companies. Keep it simple. If you were to trust the women's magazines and the department store cosmetic counters you'd think you need a shed-load of different products, according to your age, your skin type, your ethnic background. We don't agree. Skin is basically the same, whether it is dry or oily, whether it is black, white or Asian. We got so fed up with all the hype that we developed our own products and kept the line as simple as possible: just a very few really great products at sensible prices that suit all skins. Why make life more complicated than it needs to be? However, you don't remotely need to buy our creams and serum – there are plenty of other options available.

Your face regime

STEP ONE: CLEANSE

This step is totally vital, and often ignored or underplayed. But without clean skin there is very little point in piling on fancy creams and unguents. They will simply sit on top of your old make-up, dead skin and dirt. Nice, eh? Ideally you should cleanse your face and neck thoroughly twice a day, once in the morning and once before going to bed. You might be interested to know that your skin is estimated to age by a week for every night you don't remove your make-up!

- Remove all make-up. Be careful not to drag or pull the skin, especially the delicate skin around your eyes. Don't ever pick off mascara. Permanent make-up and eyebrow/lash dyeing prevent the need for so much make-up so are worth considering.

- Cleanse thoroughly. It's up to you what kind of cleanser you use, but for truly clean skin you will really need to use water at some point. If you use a wipe-off cleanser, finish with a blast of warm water to remove any oily residue. We don't advise soap, however, as it can upset the skin's natural pH balance, making it too alkaline.

- Using a flannel or washcloth gives your skin a gentle exfoliation every day, essential for renewing cells. Make sure your facecloth is soft and keep it scrupulously clean, boil-washing every few days.

- Splash your face with plenty of warm water. Toner really isn't necessary. But water is essential.

STEP TWO: MOISTURISE

Once your face and neck are perfectly clean, you can choose your moisturiser or serum of choice. This helps to lock in moisture above all, but (depending on the cream) may also squeeze skincare nutrients into your skin. We don't want to be prescriptive with which cream you choose – it will depend a lot on your individual skin and your budget. Be reassured, however, that the price of a cream does not necessarily denote how effective it is. Equally, you should not pick too heavy a cream as your skin needs to breathe and you don't want to block your pores. We'll look at specific ingredients later in the book.

In the morning you should choose a light cream or serum that is easily and quickly absorbed into your skin. We like to use one that tones the skin, giving a lifting effect. In the evening, before bed, pick a rejuvenating cream that will reduce the appearance of lines and wrinkles, getting to work while you sleep. We also suggest a dedicated eye gel or cream to safeguard the delicate skin around your eyes and to prevent lines (used both morning and night).

STEP THREE: SUNSCREEN (MORNING ONLY)

Apply sunscreen and allow to dry for about ten minutes before applying make-up.

DIY MICRODERMABRASION?

Exfoliation is a buzzword at the moment and we're seeing a lot of home 'microdermabrasion' treatments, kits and DIY peels. Be careful. Vigorous DIY exfoliation can cause a rapid thinning of the epidermis and may leave your skin irritated and sensitive to light. Your skin will automatically exfoliate in its own natural cycle every few weeks. It's actually better to go in for gentle daily exfoliation (which will occur naturally as you cleanse properly) at home. Leave the deeper work to the experts.

Your body regime

Once again, the basic regime is incredibly simple: cleanse and moisturise. However we would also advocate you diligently skin-brush – every day for best results.

STEP ONE: SKIN-BRUSH

If you want to make your body look fabulous, this really is essential. The brushing gives sluggish circulation and lymphatic systems a boost and also softens any impacted lymph mucus from your lymph nodes. It is especially useful in helping to break down cellulite. It's incredibly simple, yet incredibly effective.

Always use a pure bristle brush and dry-brush on dry skin (so *before* you get into the bath or shower).

- Start with your feet and brush all over, including the soles.

- Now brush up your legs, front and back, using smooth long strokes, always moving towards the groin area (where there are major lymph nodes). Don't scrub or press too hard – it won't work as well.

- Bottom next. You can be a bit firmer here but keep it smooth. Do your best to reach your mid-back (or ask for help), always moving towards the armpits (another major lymph site).

- Move on to your arms, from your hands (don't forget your palms) up to your armpits.

- Brush across your shoulders and down your chest towards the heart. Don't brush your nipples and be very gentle over your breasts. Brush down the back of the neck.

- Now brush your abdomen, avoiding your genitals. Use a circular movement, in a clockwise direction, as this helps to stimulate the colon.

- Be thorough and keep brushing for at least five minutes. Your skin should be glowing and you should feel wonderfully energised. Now have your bath or shower.

STEP TWO: CLEANSE

As with your face, avoid soap and use a dedicated body wash instead (most now have great active compounds to boost your skin).

STEP THREE: MOISTURISE

Use a good quality body moisturiser, packed with active ingredients to keep skin soft and supple. Always apply while your skin is slightly damp.

Remember to use sunscreen too if you are exposing your body to the sun. Hands, in particular, are often left out and can easily age with overexposure to the sun.

There you have it – your incredibly simple, hugely effective Rejuvenation Plan. Stick to it for at least six weeks and you will notice really dramatic benefits. Once you have reached that point, we can guarantee you won't want to go back to your old, skin-ageing ways.

CHAPTER FIVE

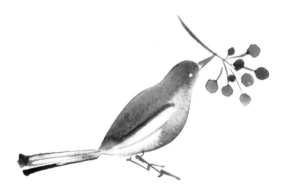

The hormone connection

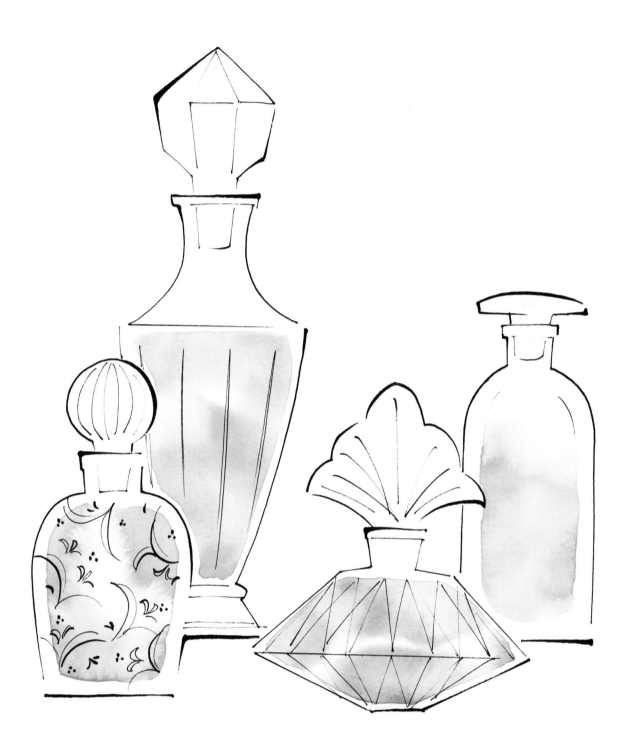

People underestimate the power of their hormones. When patients come to see us, we always keep in the back of our minds that surgery might not be the entire answer. Sometimes what is needed is hormonal rebalancing. Someone might come in wanting a breast enlargement, because she has particularly small breasts. Yes, it might just be the luck (or ill-luck) of the draw, but equally it could be because she has an imbalance in her female hormones. Similarly, someone might come in asking for LipoSelection but the reason she has large fat deposits is because her thyroid is out of balance. As doctors, we have a duty to look at all possible reasons for lack of proportion.

Why are hormones so important?

Hormones are chemicals secreted by your glands into the bloodstream in order to bring about a specific effect on tissues elsewhere in the body. The various glands that make up the hormone system combine to create an incredibly complex control and communications network, working alongside the nervous system to run the body. Many hormones are produced by the endocrine glands (the adrenals, ovaries, pituitary, pancreas and thyroid). Others are secreted from other organs, such as the kidneys, the brain, the intestines and, during pregnancy, the placenta.

Hormones affect every area of our lives: they regulate our moods, whether we feel up and happy, low and depressed, or edgy and anxious. They affect how we sleep and how much energy we have, or don't have. They are responsible for our appetite, not only for food but also for sex.

As we get older our hormone levels are often disturbed and frequently diminished. Hence the common use of HRT (hormone replacement therapy) for women going through the menopause. But few people realise that hormone imbalance can lie behind a host of symptoms beyond hot flushes and night sweats. If we want to look good throughout our lives, and offset ageing as long as possible, it's essential that we take a long hard look at our hormones.

The most common symptom of unbalanced hormone levels is fatigue. Sounds familiar? Another frequent symptom is weight gain (even when you diet and exercise your socks off). Sleep disturbances, decreased libido and depression also crop up time and time again. Feel like your memory is getting worse and worse? Might need to blame your hormones. Unable to control those sugar and carbohydrate cravings? Yes, could be hormones again.

These are all common symptoms of hormonal imbalance:

- Fatigue
- Weight gain
- Cravings for sweets, salt or carbohydrate
- Feeling depressed or overwhelmed
- Feeling anxious
- Feeling irritable
- Lack of libido/sex drive
- Insomnia or restless sleep
- Mood swings
- Hot flushes, night sweats
- PMS

- Irregular or painful periods
- Vaginal dryness
- Digestive problems
- Urinary problems
- Palpitations
- Hair loss
- Dry skin
- Premature wrinkles
- Fibroids
- Joint pains/stiffness
- Confusion, memory loss, forgetfulness

Are your hormones out of balance?

For a true picture of your hormonal health, you obviously need to have a broad spectrum of tests (a hormone panel). However, we can usually get a pretty good idea if hormones are causing havoc in your body by asking the following questions:

1   Are you on the contraceptive Pill (or have you used it regularly in the past)?
2   Have you had a hysterectomy/sterilisation?
3   Have you ever suffered from problems in your uterus, ovaries or fallopian tubes?
4   Do you have fibroids?
5   Do you have a history of fertility problems or miscarriage?
6   Do you suffer from painful, heavy or irregular periods?
7   Do you suffer from PMS?
8   Do you suffer from excessive water retention?
9   Do you have hot flushes or night sweats?
10 Do you frequently feel depressed or overwhelmed?
11 Do you have erratic mood swings?
12 Has your sex drive dropped, or has it always been low?
13 Do you suffer from anxiety or panic attacks?
14 Do you suffer from insomnia or disturbed sleep patterns?
15 Do you have more hair than normal on your body?
16 Is the hair on your head thinning?
17 Have you noticed weight gain on your thighs or hips, or around your abdomen in the last year or so?
18 Do you have cravings for sweets, sugar, salt or carbohydrate?
19 Do you often feel forgetful or confused?
20 Do you have unexplained digestive or urinary problems?

Answering yes to any of these questions may indicate your hormones are out of balance. However, it's more likely to be true if you score more than four. If you score over six, you should definitely have your hormone levels checked by a doctor.

Which hormone is to blame for your symptoms?

Tick all the symptoms you have at the moment to get a broad idea of which hormones could be out of balance. Please note this is not a substitute for clinical diagnosis, and if you think your hormones are out of balance please consult your doctor (and ideally a qualified endocrinologist – a doctor specialising in hormones).

OESTROGEN DEFICIENCY

- Tender breasts ☐
- Hot flushes ☐
- Night sweats ☐
- Low sex drive ☐
- Vaginal dryness ☐
- Incontinence ☐
- Palpitations ☐
- Aches/pains ☐
- Thinning skin ☐
- Hair loss ☐
- Depression ☐
- Disturbed sleep ☐
- Anxiety ☐
- Memory lapses ☐

OESTROGEN EXCESS

- Tender breasts ☐
- Water retention/bloating ☐
- Fibroids ☐
- Endometriosis ☐
- Headaches ☐
- Weight gain ☐
- Mood swings ☐
- Anxiety ☐
- PMS ☐
- Irritability ☐

PROGESTERONE DEFICIENCY

- Hot flushes ☐
- Night sweats ☐
- Water retention ☐
- Low sex drive ☐
- Vaginal dryness ☐
- Incontinence ☐
- Palpitations ☐
- Aches/pains ☐
- Thinning skin ☐
- Hair loss ☐
- Depression ☐
- Disturbed sleep ☐
- Anxiety ☐
- Memory lapses ☐

PROGESTERONE EXCESS

- Fatigue ☐
- Sleepiness ☐
- Depression ☐
- Breast tenderness ☐
- Low sex drive ☐
- Water retention ☐
- Bloating ☐
- Candida ☐

TESTOSTERONE (AND OTHER ANDROGENS) DEFICIENCY

- Hot flushes ☐
- Night sweats ☐
- Vaginal dryness ☐
- Incontinence ☐
- Decreased muscle ☐
- Insomnia ☐
- Thinning skin ☐
- Aches/pains ☐
- Hair loss ☐
- Thinning skin ☐
- Fibromyalgia ☐
- Depression ☐
- Memory lapses ☐
- Confusion ☐

TESTOSTERONE (AND OTHER ANDROGENS) EXCESS

- Oily skin ☐
- Acne ☐
- Excess facial hair ☐
- Loss of hair on scalp ☐
- Tender breasts ☐
- Anxiety ☐
- Anger ☐

CORTISOL DEFICIENCY

- Allergies ☐
- Asthma ☐
- Eczema ☐
- Chemical sensitivity ☐
- Muscle stiffness ☐
- Fibromyalgia ☐
- Sinusitis ☐
- Low blood pressure ☐
- Neck pain ☐
- Back pain ☐
- Arthritis ☐
- Hives ☐
- Itching ☐
- Sugar cravings ☐
- Salt cravings ☐
- Fatigue ☐
- Stress ☐

CORTISOL EXCESS

- Hot flushes ☐
- Stress ☐
- Anxiety ☐
- Fatigue ☐
- Weight gain (abdominal) ☐
- Insomnia ☐
- Sleep disturbance ☐
- Poor muscle tone ☐
- Memory lapses ☐
- Sugar cravings ☐

THYROID DEFICIENCY

Fatigue ☐
Weight gain ☐
Dizziness ☐
Joint pains/aches ☐
Muscle weakness ☐
Headaches ☐
Hair loss ☐
Swollen fingers ☐
Low body ☐
temperature

Low stamina ☐
Depression ☐
Anxiety ☐
Poor concentration ☐
Mood swings ☐
PMS ☐
Irritability ☐
Memory lapses ☐
Mixing up words ☐
Poor concentration ☐

THYROID EXCESS

Fatigue ☐
Weight loss/gain ☐
Hair loss ☐
Anaemia ☐
Rapid heartbeat ☐
Chest pain ☐
Shortness of breath ☐
Weakness ☐
Hives ☐
Itching ☐
Brittle nails ☐
Increased thirst ☐
Intolerant of heat ☐
Irregular periods ☐
Anxiety ☐
Panic attacks ☐
Depression ☐
Irritability ☐
Anger ☐
Mood swings ☐

HUMAN GROWTH HORMONE (HGH) DEFICIENCY

Poor skin quality ☐
Wrinkles ☐
Slow healing ☐
Thin skin ☐
Receding gums ☐
Sagging cheeks ☐
Abdominal fat ☐
Thinning hair ☐
Depression ☐
Fatigue ☐

Why are we unbalanced?

Hormone levels naturally fluctuate throughout our lives. For example human growth hormone, as the name suggests, is highest during our growing years and starts to tail off as we reach our thirties. All women notice their hormone levels changing as they move through their monthly cycle and we're familiar with the concept of the menopause, when hormone levels take a longer term shift. Many hormones naturally decline as we get older and there are good arguments for topping some of these up to retain their rejuvenating properties. We often refer our patients to specialists in anti-ageing hormone therapy, and we see wonderful results. However we would counsel you only to do this under medical supervision and not be tempted to self-treat. Hormones are complex chemicals and you should always consult a qualified endocrinologist rather than trying to treat yourself with individual hormones. Replacing one hormone will alter the levels of other hormones and you could end up with an even worse imbalance.

However, having said this, there are other factors that influence our hormones – factors over which we do exert some control. These include:

- Diet
- Exercise
- Pollution
- Food additives/pesticides
- Sleep
- Stress

Oestrogen dominance

In an ideal female body, the female hormones oestrogen (there are three types) and progesterone are balanced. When this happens PMS, fibroids, endometriosis, osteoporosis and the miseries of the menopause simply don't occur.

Unfortunately our modern life makes this balance virtually impossible to obtain without serious work, and oestrogen dominance (where the oestrogen/progesterone balance is disrupted) is a severe problem in our society. Synthetic oestrogens such as those in the Pill and HRT can create this imbalance, and many doctors blame the sharp rise of oestrogen-dominance on the Pill. However there are other factors to consider.

Dairy and meat products are now routinely given hormones to increase yield (along with antibiotics and other drugs) and we take these into our bodies where they affect our hormones. We also absorb an overload of xeno-oestrogens (oestrogenic chemicals in the environment). These come from a huge variety of sources: pesticides, herbicides, plastics (which can leach into food and drink), some cosmetics (watch out for the parabens group in particular) and even some food additives. These 'false' oestrogens disrupt the natural sex hormone balance. Incidentally this is also a real concern for men who are being unintentionally 'feminised' by all these xeno-oestrogens and many experts fear that we may see a huge rise in male infertility as a result. The answer is to keep away from these xeno-oestrogens as far as humanly possible (see the Good Hormone Lifestyle Plan). Some nutritional therapists also recommend using progesterone creams to balance oestrogen dominance. Consult a professional to see if this might be suitable for you.

The Good Hormone Diet Plan

1   Eat a good balanced, varied diet rich in vitamins and minerals. The interplay between hormone balance and micronutrients is complex so keep your diet as broad as possible. A nutritional therapist can tailor a diet precisely for your individual hormone imbalance: we highly recommend you consult one.

2   Eat organic whenever possible (ideally all the time). So much non-organic food is laden with pesticides and other chemicals that can affect your hormones.

3   Drink plenty of filtered (ideally reverse osmosis or carbon-filtered) water and herbal/fruit teas. NOTE: do not buy water in plastic containers as chemicals can leach into the water. Spring water in glass bottles is a suitable alternative.

4   Cut out sugar, chocolate and all refined carbohydrates. They cause energy spikes, and create imbalance in your adrenals. Artificial sweeteners should be avoided too.

5   Avoid coffee, tea, fizzy drinks and alcohol. These all interfere with your hormones.

6   Avoid hydrogenated and partially hydrogenated trans fats. These worsen hormone imbalance (in particular leading to PMS). Trans fats are usually found in most types of processed foods, especially biscuits, cakes and bread. They are also used as cooking oils for deep-frying in many restaurants and in the food industry.

7   Cut out all non-organic meat and dairy produce intake. Animals are increasingly given hormones to promote meat and dairy yield which, in turn, will interfere with your own levels.

8   Up your intake of hormone-balancing foods. Superfoods include oats, whole grains, celery, fennel, citrus fruits, rhubarb, pulses, legumes and lentils. NOTE: if your thyroid is underactive you may need advice on adapting your diet, as many of the green super-vegetables actually stimulate thyroid hormone production.

9   Consume more essential fatty acids. Eat deep-sea oily fish (salmon, fresh tuna, herring, mackerel), organic nuts and seeds (sesame, sunflower, flax, pumpkin). Use a high quality broad-spectrum omega oil (ideally omega-3, -6 and -9) for your salad dressings (Udo's Choice is excellent). Consider supplements if you cannot increase your intake.

10   Ensure you get enough B vitamins, magnesium and zinc. These vitamins and minerals have been shown to help balance hormone levels. Boost your diet with whole grains, nuts, seeds, green vegetables, root vegetables and seaweed. Try supplementing with a good quality B complex (containing 100–200mg of B6) and a multi-mineral that contains 200–400mg of magnesium and 20mg of zinc. A nutritional therapist can give you an individually tailored programme of supplements.

Consider whey

New research suggests that whey, the by-product of milk, could be a serious contender for hormonal superfood of the moment. Whey seems to impact on a wide number of hormones – and all for the best. It improves insulin sensitivity, moderates the stress hormone cortisol and boosts serotonin (the feelgood chemical). It also appears to help you lose weight and turn flab to muscle. Researchers are focusing in particular on whey's effect on the hormone cholecystokinin, a regulator of appetite that is secreted by the gut.

Add to that the fact it boosts levels of key immune-enhancing chemicals and antioxidants and it's clear that whey is the way to go.

You can buy whey powder from health shops and add it to porridge or smoothies.

The Good Hormone Lifestyle Plan

1   Find ways of dealing with stress. Excess stress plays havoc with hormone levels. Figure out a way of keeping stress under control that works for you.

2   Exercise regularly. Don't be tempted to over-exercise, however, as this can unbalance hormonal levels.

3   Sort out sleep. It's a bit of a vicious circle really: if you don't sleep well, your hormone levels will be disrupted; but if your hormones levels are out of sync, you won't sleep well. However, you can help your hormones by doing all you can to optimise sleep.

4   Avoid plastic containers and wrapping for food as the chemical compounds found in plastic can disrupt hormone levels. Use glass containers for heating food, buy food without plastic wrappings if possible (or if impossible transfer it immediately on returning home).

5   Avoid dry-cleaning if you possibly can. If not, take clothes out of the plastic wrapping the moment you get home and hang them outside to outgas for at least two hours.

6   Cut out household chemicals in your life. Switch to natural alternatives for cleaning, washing, washing up and so on (products such as Ecover offer good alternatives) or check your health shop.

7   Make your home a chemical-free zone. Modern paints, floorings, furniture, soft furnishings, bed linen and so forth are packed full of chemicals that can affect your hormones – and your general health. Choose natural untreated materials wherever possible. There are now many organic and chemical-free decorating materials available. Consider, too, recycled or antique furniture.

8   Go green in your garden. Many pesticides and herbicides disrupt your hormones. Garden organically as far as you can.

9   If you are on the Pill, consider alternatives. There are plenty of contraceptive choices that don't involve messing with your hormones. Discuss it with your doctor. If you are on HRT, consider alternatives. Many women manage the symptoms solely using diet, herbs and supplements – see a nutritional therapist or medical herbalist. Bioidentical hormones can also offer a safer approach (see page 76).

10   Cultivate good emotional health. While our hormones influence our emotions, our emotions also affect our hormones. Our hormonal system is often seen as a bridge between mind and body – the emotional and the physical. Nurture yourself, be kind to yourself, foster good relationships, take time out.

Herbal help for your hormones

Certain herbs have wonderful hormone-balancing properties. If you would like to investigate this route, we would recommend you consult a well-qualified medical herbalist who can prescribe a personalised mix of herbs. These are the most commonly prescribed.

- Agnus castus: traditionally used to relieve premenstrual and menopausal symptoms. It is high in oestrogenic plant steroids (but don't worry, these naturally occurring oestrogens actually balance the female hormones, unlike synthetic ones). It also encourages the pituitary to control excess secretion of prolactin. NOTE: be careful if you are taking the Pill – agnus castus may counteract its effects.

- Black cohosh: a well-respected natural alternative to HRT that can give relief from hot flushes and vaginal dryness. Black cohosh lowers luteinising hormone (LH) and generally balances the female sex hormones. It also has a very calming effect on the adrenals.

- Bladderwrack (kelp): supports the thyroid, useful in cases of underactive thyroid and may help with weight problems associated with this condition. Also stimulates the metabolism.

- Dandelion: a powerful diuretic, useful in cases of water retention. A natural source of potassium. Dandelion also has the intriguing ability to clear up excess hormones, in particular oestrogen.

- Ginseng (panax ginseng): an adaptogen (balancing) herb that supports the adrenals and sex hormones in particular. NOTE: avoid during pregnancy and avoid caffeine when taking.

- Liquorice: an adaptogen that has a marked effect on the hormones, in particular balancing the sex and adrenal hormones. Liquorice is clever in that it will lower your oestrogen levels when they are too high and increase them when they are too low. NOTE: do not use liquorice if you are pregnant or have high blood pressure.

- Red clover: contains isoflavones, natural plant oestrogens that balance female hormones.

- Siberian ginseng (eleutherococcus): a superb adaptogenic tonic, useful for balancing the adrenals in particular.

- Wild yam: rich in diosgenin, a precursor of progesterone, so helps to balance the female hormones. It is also important in regulating adrenal function. Some herbalists prescribe a combination of wild yam with fenugreek to increase the size of your breasts.

Bioidentical hormone therapy

Bioidentical hormones are manufactured so that they have precisely the same molecular structure as the natural hormones secreted in your own body. Synthetic hormones, on the other hand, have a different structure, basically so drug companies can patent them; typical brands include the HRT drugs Premarin and Provera.

As many women have found, synthetic hormones can produce side effects and may carry some health risks. While no exceedingly long-term studies have been conducted into bioidentical hormones, they appear to be much safer than synthetic hormones. They are a natural form and our bodies can metabolise them in a totally natural way. However, we must point out, they *are* a drug treatment.

Bioidentical hormones aren't new but what *is* new is the way many endocrinologists are now using them. In the past, patients have usually been given a one-size-fits-all dose which, to our mind, is pretty much the same as giving generic synthetic HRT. Now, however, an individualised approach is common. If hormone imbalance is suspected, you will be given a batch of laboratory tests to determine your hormone levels (known as a hormone panel). This will tell the doctor exactly which hormones you need supplementing, and in which dosages. For example, you could be prescribed a combination of estradiol (one of the forms of oestrogen), testosterone, progesterone and DHEA. Your combination is then made up at the pharmacy and your progress would be monitored closely (usually you could expect to have your tests repeated every three months or so). Once the optimum balance is achieved, testing would be reduced to about once a year.

We feel that if your symptoms do not respond to the natural hormone balancing plans then bioidentical hormone therapy is a good route to follow.

DHEA: taking on abdominal fat?

DHEA (dehydroepiandrosterone) is a steroid hormone produced by the adrenal glands, the ovaries and the brain that is essential for the production of other hormones, including oestrogen and testosterone. DHEA levels peak in our mid-twenties and then drop off as we get older. Low levels seem to equate with all the signs of ageing: increased heart disease, excess body fat, decreased muscle mass.

The exact effect DHEA has on the body's cells isn't completely clear but what does seem certain is that when we supplement it in older people, they report feeling a much greater sense of well-being – and they tend to lose weight. Recent studies show that DHEA significantly reduced abdominal fat and improved insulin action. It also seems likely that DHEA can boost the immune system and may even protect against osteoporosis, high cholesterol and heart disease.

A study into DHEA at the University of California Medical School found that men and women between the ages of forty and seventy who took 50mg of DHEA a day for six months reported feeling more relaxed, sleeping better and handling stress better.

You can buy DHEA over the counter, but it's best to take it under the auspices of a doctor. Too much DHEA can cause side effects such as facial hair while many OTC supplements simply don't have enough DHEA to make any significant difference. We think it's a powerful anti-ageing supplement and often recommend it to our patients.

Human Growth Hormone (HGH): the miracle youth hormone

HGH is being touted as a youth elixir, a miracle rejuvenating substance that could offset many of the symptoms of ageing. Originally it was used purely for children who didn't grow as anticipated. However now attention is being turned on HGH as a superb anti-ageing tool. HGH levels start to decline from the ages of twenty-five to thirty and by the time we reach middle age many of us are seriously low in HGH.

As you'll see from the checklist of symptoms for HGH deficiency, virtually all the markers of ageing are there, in particular all the wrinkles, sagging skin and increased body fat that we are trying to avoid. Research shows great benefits for HGH therapy, both physical and mental. When HGH injections are given, these are common results:

- Decrease in body fat (15 per cent on average and up to 50 per cent reduction of abdominal fat)
- Increased bone density
- Increased aerobic (cardiovascular) capacity
- Increased energy
- Increased strength
- Increased muscle
- Improved memory
- Improved concentration
- Brighter mood
- Better sleep patterns
- Reduction of wrinkles
- Thicker, plumper skin
- More lustrous hair

Basically you can turn yourself from flabby, frail, wrinkled and lethargic to energy-charged, smoother skinned and much smarter. It's very tempting, isn't it?

Some people, however, do notice side effects which can include:

- Oedema (swelling) particularly in hands
- Carpal tunnel syndrome
- Joint pain
- Mild numbness
- Elevated glucose levels (rare)

Contraindications: HGH should not be used for patients who are diabetic or who have active cancer.

Should you try HGH? At the moment it's an expensive treatment and you would require regular injections, regular medical supervision and regular blood tests. However, it's certainly worth having your levels tested once you hit your forties. There is no benefit in supplementing HGH while your own levels are still good. At present HGH is not licensed as an anti-ageing drug but we consider it a strong pillar in anti-ageing medicine.

CHAPTER SIX

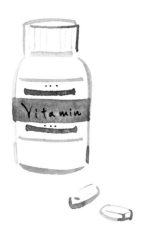

Preparing for surgery

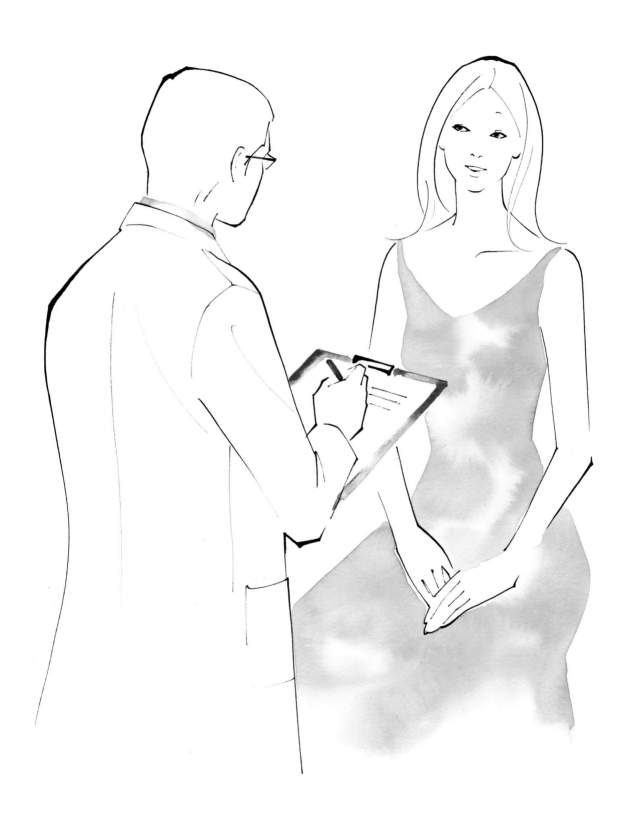

Before you even think about surgery, we would ask you to swear to us, hand on heart, that you have read, taken in and (most importantly) carried out the advice in all the chapters up to this point. Truly, it will save you a lot of time and money in consultation fees. You need to be absolutely clear about why you want surgery and what you expect it will do for you. The biggest mistake people make is having unrealistic expectations. This applies as much for non-invasive procedures as for invasive surgery. We say time and time again that while cosmetic surgery can give you a huge boost of self-esteem, it cannot change your life all by itself. You need to be 100, 150, per cent certain that you are having surgery for the right reasons. Once you are quite sure, then you need to prepare.

The Two Vital Steps you must take before surgery

1   **Get your weight down**: if you are overweight you really do need to spend the time and effort to lose those extra pounds before having surgery. Any good surgeon will not accept you for body contouring or fat removal if you have too much weight to lose. Follow the eating and exercise advice we have already given. Even if you are not having surgery specifically aimed at the fat deposits, it's still a good idea to be as near your ideal weight as possible, since being overweight is a risk factor for any surgery.

2   **Stop smoking**: there is very little point having cosmetic surgery if you are going to continue to smoke. Not only does it make your surgery more risk-prone but it will also undo all our best efforts to make you look younger. Smoking is contraindicated for most major surgery; a good surgeon will simply refuse to work on you unless you give up. Talk to your doctor about the easiest way to quit.

How to find your surgeon

There are many excellent surgeons out there, there truly are. However, sadly, there are also many who are not so good. As the appeal of cosmetic surgery grows, many doctors have seen it as a lucrative proposition and have moved into the field without what we consider adequate training and experience. The situation is better than it used to be: in the past, there were no regulations to prevent any doctor from setting up in cosmetic surgery without training or experience. During the past few years some regulations have been introduced to ensure that surgeons do at least undergo some training and that clinics have reasonable standards. However the situation is still quite foggy and we are not satisfied with the way the industry is regulated. In the future we hope there will be a comprehensive policy that governs all of Europe. We also feel there should be a graduate-level university or centre for training in cosmetic surgery.

In the meantime, you have to be very wise and smart, and do some serious homework before you trust your face or body to a surgeon.

We would strongly advise you to limit your choice to those surgeons who are registered with the organisations listed in the Resources section of this book (BAAPS, BAPS, etc.), which will ensure they have, at least, been trained to a minimum standard. It is not, however, an assurance of excellence. Also ensure your surgeon works within a clinic recognised by the Healthcare Commission (see Resources), which will guarantee that the clinic has been vetted and passed. Your choice is a personal one too. Unfortunately it's not quite the done thing to go up to a woman in the gym and ask who did her face or her lipo! It's one thing asking for the name of a hairdresser but blatantly asking for her cosmetic surgeon could seriously offend (even if she did disappear for a couple of weeks and come back looking twenty years younger). Your GP, dentist or gynaecologist might be able to suggest good surgeons, as could friends and relatives who have had cosmetic surgery. You might have read about certain people in magazines or papers. You may have seen adverts (though we have to say that most really good surgeons never need to advertise). Gather all this information together in your file – the more information you have, the better.

Send off for brochures from the clinics you like the sound of; visit their websites and check the surgeons' credentials. While long years of experience are usually a good thing, you need to be sure that your surgeon has kept up to date with the latest procedures and advances – and hasn't become a fossil.

Costs

Cosmetic surgery is not cheap. It is a large investment and so you need to be sure you will get value for money. However, while it's tempting to take the cheapest surgery on offer, it may not be a wise move. Equally, picking the most expensive does not guarantee the best results. You need the right surgeon for the right procedure for you, and you alone. We're often asked if it's possible to have surgery free of charge. Wouldn't it be great if you could get your body perfected on the NHS? Sadly, it's highly unlikely. However there are some cases in which your doctor will recommend you for surgery, and the NHS will pick up the bill. Breast reduction (where the breasts are very heavy and causing postural problems) is one example. Ask your GP – it's worth a try.

Before you schedule your first consultation: the vital checklist

You can save yourself a lot of time, money and effort by fine-tuning your list of potential surgeons. There is no point in having a consultation with a surgeon who does not perform the procedure you want, or whose fees you cannot afford. Before you even go to see the surgeon these are the ten questions you need to ask:

1 Is the clinic registered with the Healthcare Commission?

2 Is the surgeon a specialist in cosmetic surgery? What qualifications do they have? What training have they undergone? How long have they been practising cosmetic surgery? What percentage of their practice is devoted to cosmetic surgery? (Avoid someone who has done a brief weekend course or only performs a few surgeries a year.) Are they registered with BAAPS or BAPS?

3 Are they experienced in the procedure you want? It's no good going to an expert in rhinoplasty if you're after a superb tummy tuck and they only do one in a blue moon.

4 Does the clinic offer the procedures you want? While most clinics cover a wide range of procedures, they do vary in their specialities and preferences.

5 Does the clinic offer the most up-to-date advances and procedures? It makes sense to have a choice of the least invasive and most effective procedures. We make a point of going to all the major conferences and acquire new training all the time – your surgeon should too.

6   How much will your procedure cost? Can you afford it? Check that you are given total costs (including any possible extras).

7   Does the clinic practise from a hospital or have hospital privileges? This ensures that, if necessary, you can be transferred to a hospital with your surgeon in attendance. It's vital, particularly for more invasive procedures. All major surgery that requires general anaesthesia and an overnight stay should be carried out in a hospital.

8   How long is your consultation likely to take and how much will it cost? Most clinics only charge one consultation fee, regardless of how many times you come back before your procedure. Consultations can vary between fifteen minutes and an hour – obviously the longer the better.

9   Will the consultation be with your surgeon? Amazingly, some clinics fob you off with someone other than the surgeon. We strongly advise against this; only a surgeon can assess your suitability for surgery.

10 Where is the clinic based? If you will have to travel remember to factor in transport costs and any hotel stays that might be necessary. Ensure you will have someone to take you home after surgery. If you have sedation you are not legally allowed to drive or travel on public transport for forty-eight hours after surgery.

Your first consultation

By now you should have a shortlist of surgeons. We would recommend that, however tempting it may be to race in, you should see several consultants before making your final decision. The 'very best' surgeon your friend swears by might not be the right person for you. A clinic that looks great on paper or on its website might not feel so reassuring in the flesh. Cosmetic surgery is a serious business and it's essential you feel totally comfortable with your surgeon and the place in which they practise. Ultimately it's a very personal decision. What feels right for you? Who feels right to you? Again, we would stress this is a partnership: we need to work together with our patients, and all good surgeons will tell you exactly the same thing. If you feel intimidated or uncomfortable with your surgeon, it won't be a good partnership. You won't feel free to ask the questions you need to ask. You might not end up with the result you want. While the first part of the process is all about facts, the second part will probably also bring in intuition. Yes, you need to know your surgeon can do the procedure and do it well but, over and above that, do you get a good feeling from them?

Remember to go to your appointments well prepared. Take your notebook and your list of questions. Write down the answers to your questions; with the best will in the world, you won't remember everything after the appointment unless you do.

Having consulted with several doctors, you should have narrowed your choice down to two or three. Go back and see your first choice again. Do you still feel comfortable? Is your memory correct? Are you happy to put your face or body in their hands? It's natural to feel nervous about surgery, but you should never go into cosmetic surgery feeling nervous about your surgeon.

What to ask your surgeon: the ten vital questions

1   Am I a good candidate for this procedure? There are many factors that can affect the result you will get from surgery, including your skin type and how elastic it is; your bone structure; your general health and fitness; whether you have had previous surgery in that area; your age. It's vital to understand the limitations of any surgical procedure.

2   Is this the best procedure for the effect I want? Although you may know which procedure you want (maybe because you know someone who has had it, or seen before and after pictures of it in a magazine) it may not be the best choice for your skin. Your surgeon should give you options, including what they think would be the most effective choice.

3   Can you achieve the effect I want? If you explain precisely what you are looking for, your surgeon should be able to tell you if this is realistic or not. This is a vital step and you and your surgeon need to be able to agree on what can, and can't, be done.

4   What will happen before, during and after the procedure? You need to feel comfortable with all the steps of the procedure. We can give you guidelines in this book but they are based on our practice, and every surgeon works slightly differently.

5   What are the risks and complications associated with this procedure? How often have you seen them happen and what do you do to minimise them? It's important that you should not sign any medical waiver that you don't understand.

6   How long will it take before I see results? How long will my recovery take and what should I expect while it is happening? Do remember many procedures are major surgery and can entail long recovery periods. Often you may look worse before you look better – you may need patience.

7   Can I see before and after photos of recent patients who have undergone the same procedure I'm seeking? Can I talk to someone who's recently had the procedure? Of course, a clinic isn't likely to give you details of someone who was miserable with their result, but you will get some honest 'how it felt and how I feel about the results' feedback. It's also good to talk to someone who has actually experienced the procedure, as opposed to someone who performs it.

8   What should I do to prepare for this surgery? Are there lifestyle changes I need to make?

9   Do you have hospital privileges? If something goes wrong, will I automatically be transferred to a hospital where you can practise?

10 What happens if the results are not what we agreed upon? Will you undertake to redo my surgery? Will follow-up procedures cost me more?

What *not* to ask your surgeon

Some questions you should ask the surgeon's secretary, not your surgeon.

1 **Fees:** how much and what they include. Are there any extras? The quote should be all-inclusive. Ask for a breakdown so you can clearly understand what you are paying for.

2 **Payment:** when you will need to pay; what types of payment are accepted. Many clinics will ask for the cost of your consultation to be paid on the day of your initial visit. Others will include it in your final bill. Some clinics offer credit plans: check how much you will be paying in interest – you might get a better deal by shopping around for a loan. Payment is usually always in advance.

3 **Scheduling surgery:** the timetable of your operation.

The risk factors

We love cosmetic surgery and the results it can give. But it's easy, in all the excitement of thinking about your new look, to forget that many procedures require major invasive surgery. Just because cosmetic surgery is now incredibly common doesn't mean that there aren't risks. In the hands of a good surgeon these risks are, admittedly, small, and serious complications are rare, but we must point out that no surgeon can guarantee 100 per cent risk-free surgery. There may also be side effects and discomfort. Without wanting to be alarmist, it is essential you go into surgery with all the facts and it is only right and ethical that we point out what can happen if surgery goes wrong.

The major risks from cosmetic surgery are exactly the same as those you would expect from any surgery. Do remember many of these are rare and extreme:

- Temporary paralysis
- Nerve damage
- Blood clot possibly leading to stroke or embolism
- Bleeding, haematoma
- Brain damage
- Airway obstruction
- Abnormal heart rhythm
- Heart attack
- Excessive scarring
- Puckering or dimpling of the skin
- Perforation of internal organs
- Post-operative numbness
- Infection

We will discuss the possible risks and side effects of individual procedures later in the book, alongside the general information for each operation.

How can you minimise your risks?

While no one can predict unforeseen problems during or after surgery, there are certain things you can – and should – do to minimise the possibility of risks.

1   Really do your homework before surgery. Make sure you find the right surgeon for the procedure – someone with plenty of experience and good qualifications. Your surgeon should be a specialist in cosmetic surgery, not someone who just does the odd procedure. Equally, ask how many operations they will perform in a day. At some large clinics, surgeons perform far too many procedures and you shouldn't run the risk of being ninth or tenth in line as the risks will increase. Surgeons are like airline pilots – they should not work overly long hours.

2   Prepare thoroughly. It's vital to go into surgery in the best possible state of health you can: as we say, time and time again, this might involve losing weight or getting fitter.

3   Tell your surgeon your full medical history. If you have any allergies your surgeon needs to know (medications, latex, plasters, etc.). If you are on medication (such as HRT, blood thinners, anti-depressants, the Pill), you must tell your surgeon as they could affect your surgery. Also do tell your surgeon if you suffer from high blood pressure.

4   Stop taking over-the-counter medications such as aspirin for a month before surgery (discuss this with your surgeon or GP who could offer alternatives). Talk to your doctor about diuretics and diet pills too.

5   Check out your natural medicine cabinet. Some natural supplements are a no-no before and after cosmetic surgery (usually because they thin the blood too much): vitamin E, garlic and ginseng are all contraindicated, for example (see the fuller list on page 91). Tell your surgeon which supplements and herbs you take.

6   Be honest about your habits. If you take – or have taken – recreational drugs, you must come clean and tell your surgeon. They aren't there to judge and this is vital information.

7   Take the opportunity to quit smoking. Most surgeons will refuse to operate if you're a smoker. It's for your own safety. It is well known that smoking causes narrowing of the blood vessels, leading to a decreased blood supply to your skin. This, in turn, slows and interferes with the healing process.

8   Cut down on the alcohol. It's well worth taking a slow steady detox before you have cosmetic surgery as excessive alcohol intake is a risk factor.

9   Find out your family health history and share it with your surgeon. A family history of heart or lung disease, blood clots or bad reactions to anaesthetics is vital information for your surgeon.

10 Don't insist on too much cosmetic surgery in one go. This is real life, not a makeover show! Be guided by your surgeon on how much fat to have taken out during LipoSelection, or how many procedures you can have at one time – the longer you're under general anaesthetic, the more risk there is. Err on the side of caution; remember, you can always have more done later.

When not to have surgery

Not everyone should undertake cosmetic surgery. You should not have surgery if:

1   You have unrealistic expectations or if you are seeking perfection.

2   You think cosmetic surgery will magically transform your life.

3   You are going through divorce or experiencing a rocky time in your relationship.

4   You have just suffered a trauma – a bereavement, loss of job, accident.

5   You have a mental illness, any form of psychosis or paranoia.

6   You have an eating disorder.

7   You suffer from body dysmorphic disorder (BDD).

8   You are under exceptional stress.

9   You are physically or emotionally run-down.

10 You are suffering from depression or extreme anxiety.

This may sound draconian but there are good reasons for these contraindications.

You need to be in a position to make good, healthy, clear-headed choices about cosmetic surgery. You need to be well-balanced, calm and reasoned about what you want and why you want it.

It's never a good idea to make life-changing choices when you are out of balance. Nobody who is stressed, depressed or traumatised – for whatever reason – is in a good place to decide on surgical procedures. You need to take the time to get back on an even keel. You may need to seek help from a psychiatrist, psychologist or counsellor. Relationship counselling, sex therapy or bereavement counselling could be called for. You might just need to cut down on your overload, find ways to control your stress and improve your sleep. You need to talk to your GP about how best to deal with depression or anxiety.

Balanced choices only come from a balanced mind. Don't race into cosmetic surgery – there is nothing to be lost by waiting a few months or even years. In fact, the way advances are forging ahead, you might benefit from a newer, better procedure if you wait a little.

Body dysmorphia and cosmetic surgery

One group of people in particular should not seek cosmetic surgery under any circumstances, and that's people suffering from body dysmorphic disorder (BDD). BDD is an obsessive/compulsive psychiatric condition that centres around an uncontrollable preoccupation with any defect (whether slight or purely imagined) in your appearance. The focus can be on any part of the body but most people with BDD are worried about more than one area.

People with BDD usually:

- Spend from three to eight hours a day worrying about their physical flaws.

- Frequently and obsessively check their appearance in the mirror.

- Constantly ask other people about their appearance, seeking reassurance.

- Try to camouflage the troubling part of the body by wearing lots of layers of clothing, excessive make-up or hats.

- Suffer low self-esteem.

- Suffer depression.

- Self-harm to some degree.

Anyone suffering from BDD is not a good candidate for surgery. You would inevitably be dissatisfied with the result – however successful – and experience shows that distress may actually increase following surgery, or you might simply become preoccupied with a different part of the body.

BDD can be treated: cognitive behavioural therapy (CBT) and antidepressant medication have produced good results. Consult your GP.

The Top Ten Total Disasters

You can spot them a mile off: women who have simply had too much or gone too far. Choose the wrong surgeon or insist on too much extreme surgery and one of these could be the result.

1 The Wind Tunnel: overly tight facelifts that give the dreaded Mach Ten effect.

2 The Trout Pout: way too much filler or oversized implants make you look as if you have had an accident with a door.

3 The Hamster: oversized or badly positioned implants on the cheeks or chin.

4 The Cat's Eyes: too much lateral pull or too many upper facelifts give that unpleasant Bride of Wildenstein look.

5 The Over-peel: where you end up with shiny, gleaming white skin that doesn't remotely match your neck, hands and décolleté.

6 The Shocked Brow: that awful startled 'What, are you looking at *me*?!' look when the brow is overlifted.

7 The Michael Jackson Nose: in other words, overdone and out of proportion. If the tips are pinched and you see right up into the nostrils, it's not a good nose.

8 The Baywatch Boob Job: massively out of proportion breasts, particularly on very slight women.

9 The Wide-apart Pair: spherical breasts plonked wide apart on the chest – unnatural and unsightly.

10 The Bionic Bottom: again, out of proportion bouncy buttocks on tiny-framed women.

Timetable of surgery: which surgery when?
What to have done at each age

Everyone ages at different rates. You could have inherited great skin and a fabulous metabolism from your parents, or you could have drawn the short genetic straw. Equally your lifestyle can affect how you look. Eating, drinking and smoking habits can pave the way for poor skin, as can excessive stress, poor sleep and overexposure to the sun and wind. However, it's possible to give a rough idea of what kind of problems are associated with each age bracket and what can be done more effectively at each stage of your life.

AGE	PROBLEM	PROCEDURE TO FIX
Mid-20s-mid-30s	Frown lines	Botulinum
	Fat deposits (localised)	LipoSelection
	Breasts too small	Breast implants
	Breasts too large	Breast reduction
	Asymmetrical breasts	LipoSelection/breast implants
Mid-30s-mid-40s	Loss of tone/sagging breasts	Breast lift/implants
	Wrinkles around eyes	Botulinum/skin resurfacing
	Frown lines	Botulinum
	Wrinkles around lips	Resurfacing/peels/fillers
	Folds or creases between nose and lips	Fillers
	Hooding of eyelids	Upper eyelid surgery or brow lift
	Puffy eyes	Lower eyelid surgery
	Fat deposits, usually in hips, thighs, abdomen	LipoSelection
	Loose abdominal skin	Tummy tuck/mini tuck
	Post-baby sagging and bagging	Tummy tuck/mini tuck
		LipoSelection/breast lift
	Jowls	Contour thread lift
Mid-40s-mid-50s	Thinning lips	Fillers
	Double chin	LipoSelection
	Sagging eyebrows	Brow lift
	Jowls	MACS lift
	Looseness of facial skin/descent of cheek fat	Facelift, implants, fillers
	Crepey neck or cords in neck	Neck lift/tightening
Mid-50s and beyond	Wrinkles and creases	Resurfacing/ peels/ fat injections/ botulinum/ fillers
	Facial sagging and laxity	Repeat facelift
	'Batwing' arms	Upper arm lift

Multiple procedures: good or bad?

It often happens: you go to see a surgeon wanting a simple brow lift and the next thing you know you're being told you also need a facelift, neck lift, botulinum and a pile of resurfacing. Or you decide on a breast augmentation only to be told you'll need a breast lift too. Are you being conned? Not necessarily. Often, in order to get the very best effect, you need more than one procedure. It's a little like when you decorate a room. Once you've painted the walls, you realise the windows also need doing, and the flooring is a bit ropey, and the lighting is out of date too. While it's obviously not great to have procedures for the sake of it (and we're wary of the number of procedures done en masse on the television makeover shows) it can make surgical, and financial, sense to combine some. Why put yourself through more anaesthetic and recovery time than strictly necessary? Why pay for separate procedures spaced apart when you could save money by combining them (most surgeons will give a discount for several procedures carried out at the same time)? It's worth considering, worth keeping an open mind, if your surgeon suggests reasonable combination work.

Surgery abroad and makeover holidays

It sounds so tempting, doesn't it? You tell everyone you're off for a bit of sun, jump on a plane, and then come back a week or so later with much more than a fresh tan – in fact a whole new face and body. It seems to make perfect sense: prices are very competitive in overseas surgeries so you might be able to afford several procedures for the price of one or two here in Britain. You can rest and recuperate somewhere sunny with no need to worry about everyday life. Equally, there's absolutely no need to explain to everyone that you're going to have surgery – you're just off on holiday.

Yes, it sounds great, but we would beg you to think very long and hard about doing it. In fact, we would really much rather you didn't opt for a cosmetic surgery 'holiday' at all (and our colleagues would all agree). Aha, you're probably thinking, well you *would* say that, wouldn't you? It's in your interest for people to have surgery in this country, isn't it? Truly, we have more clients than we can cope with and have to turn people away every day. Our concern is for your health. These are the reasons why we say No, Non, Nein and Niet to sun, sea and surgery.

1   It is much tougher to check out the training and credentials of doctors overseas.
     We're not saying there aren't good surgeons abroad – of course there are. But there is
     no international standard for quality and you could undergo a procedure with a
     doctor who is poorly trained or lacking in experience.

2   You will not have the opportunity to make a shortlist of surgeons and visit them all
     prior to your trip. Most likely you won't even meet your surgeon prior to surgery.

3   The clinic in which you have your surgery may not meet adequate safety standards.
     You may not have the fall-back option of being taken to hospital should something
     go wrong during surgery.

4   You may not have the follow-up care you require after your surgery. A good surgeon
     will want to check up on the surgery and monitor your progress. This is impossible
     if you have flown home after the procedure.

5   If you have any problems after your surgery, you won't easily be able to return to your surgeon for revisions or other treatment. You may have to pay again for a revision by a UK surgeon – but be warned, many are uneasy handling this kind of revision work.

And a couple of more general points which may help you make your decision.

1   You won't be able to sunbathe. Most procedures demand you keep out of the sun until you are totally healed. So you can kiss goodbye to the idea of lazing on the beach.

2   Any kind of activity is a no-no. Most procedures require serious rest while you're recuperating. So anything active is out – that includes swimming, watersports, golf, riding, hiking, tennis and sailing. Is it really going to be fun sitting and watching everyone else enjoy themselves?

Of course, there is one exception to this rule: if your surgeon also practises in your home country then you should be fine, as they will be available for follow-ups and to sort out any glitches, should they occur.

The pre-assessment health check

All good clinics will expect you to have a full health check before scheduling surgery.

A full medical history will be taken and if you need any tests these will be arranged by the clinic. Expect to be asked about:

- General health and fitness
- Any medical problems
- Heart disease
- Lung disease
- Pain in the chest during exercise or at rest
- Diabetes
- Your current medication
- Any allergies
- Smoking
- Alcohol intake
- Support; the help you have at home

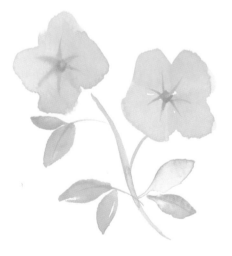

Which anaesthetic?

Anaesthetic simply means 'loss of sensation'; it's how we bring about a painless state so you don't feel any discomfort during your procedure. We use different forms of anaesthetic for varying purposes and procedures. However, often you may be given a choice. There are advantages and disadvantages to each form. Let's take a look.

IV (INTRAVENOUS) SEDATION

- What it is: the use of drugs to depress the central nervous system, putting you into a state of very deep relaxation. You will not be asleep and will be able to listen to your surgeon and nurses (and respond if requested); however you will not remember what happened afterwards. Most people find it a pleasant experience. Drugs are administered via an intravenous (into the vein) drip, usually by an anaesthetist.

- How long does it last? Usually two or three hours (although it can last up to four hours).

- Advantages: patients recover more quickly from IV sedation than general anaesthetic, and can usually go home on the same day. You can continue to take prescribed medicines and can eat and drink as normal.

- Not recommended if: you cannot lie flat; you have an illness (e.g. Parkinson's) that makes being still difficult; you have a cough you can't control; you are claustrophobic; you have severe hearing difficulties; you have breathing problems; you have difficulty understanding what is being said.

LOCAL ANAESTHETIC

- What it is: a drug that stops you feeling any pain in and around the area being treated. You will stay awake and aware of everything that is happening but you will not feel any pain. Local anaesthetic is given in the form of an injection to the area being treated.

- How long does it last? Usually two or three hours (although it can last up to four hours). It is often combined with IV sedation.

- Advantages: local anaesthetic works really well and offers pain relief after the operation as well. It has fewer risks and side effects than a general anaesthetic as it does not affect any other part of your body (such as your heart or lungs). People recover more quickly following local anaesthetic and can go home on the same day. You can continue to take any prescribed medicine and can eat and drink as normal.

- Not recommended if: you cannot lie flat; you have an illness (e.g. Parkinson's) that makes being still difficult; you have a cough you can't control; you are claustrophobic; you have severe hearing difficulties; you have breathing problems; you have difficulty understanding what is being said. It is also not advised if you suffer from anxiety, if you are very squeamish or if the operation will last over one hour.

- What it is: a combination of drugs that provoke and maintain a complete loss of consciousness, keeping you totally unaware of what is happening during your operation. Painkilling drugs are also administered by the anaesthetist so you feel no pain after surgery.

- How long does it last? General anaesthetic can be controlled very precisely by the anaesthetist and your anaesthetic will be maintained until your surgery is over.

- Advantages: you need know absolutely nothing about your operation. Allows you to stay completely still for a long period of time. Allows surgery to take place in widely separated areas of the body at the same time. Makes no psychological demands on you. Side effects are far rarer than in the past (you may have a little nausea or discomfort from lying in one position). Many operations with general anaesthetic can now be considered day cases, with you able to leave the hospital the same day as your operation.

- Not recommended if: you smoke; you've had a previous poor reaction to anaesthesia; you are extremely obese. Breathing difficulties may occur if you have a very small or receding jaw, a short neck, limited neck extension or tumours of the face, mouth, neck or throat.

Your pre-surgery diet plan

Good nutrition is vital both before and after surgery. It helps your body to prepare for the procedure and also to recuperate from it. Hopefully you will already be eating an excellent diet, as outlined previously. If not, now's the time to start. In a nutshell, follow these key points:

- Include organic low-fat protein (poultry, fish, game, etc.) with every meal. Soy products are useful too. Adequate protein is vital for wounds to heal properly.

- Include whole grains and legumes for fibre and a large amount of fresh (ideally organic) fruits and vegetables.

- Avoid 'empty' calories from junk foods, fast food, sugar, sweets and chocolate. Avoid foods high in saturated fat, hydrogenated fat and trans fat. All of these can stop your wound healing as well as it might.

- Cut out, or reduce, your caffeine intake both before and after surgery. Caffeine can interfere with wound healing.

- Cut out alcohol – it may make your surgery more risky.

Your pre-op supplement plan

If you are going to have surgery, or pretty well any procedure other than non-invasive treatments, you should prepare your body by giving it optimum doses of vital micronutrients. This will boost the immune system and help your body withstand the stress of surgery. Start taking your supplements several weeks before surgery. This is what we recommend:

1   A high quality multivitamin (take in the morning).

2   A high quality multi-mineral (take late afternoon).

3   Extra vitamin C (up to 2g a day, depending on bowel tolerance; basically, if your stools become very loose, you need to lower your dosage): take this in split doses for maximum effect. Vitamin C and zinc (below) are both vital for forming healthy collagen to repair wounds.

4   Extra zinc if necessary (check levels on your multis and antioxidants): you need 30g a day.

5   An antioxidant complex (with flavonoids): to boost your body's immune system and help to limit scarring.

6   A broad-spectrum amino acid complex: to help with tissue rebuilding.

7   Probiotics (beneficial bacteria): choose a broad-spectrum one to counteract the effect of antibiotics on the good bacteria of your gut.

8   Siberian ginseng: a fabulous adaptogenic herb that helps the body withstand stress; 200mg daily. NOTE: do not confuse this with other forms of ginseng (e.g. Panax ginseng) which should be avoided near to surgery.

IMPORTANT NOTE: check the labels of your supplements carefully. You must not take any more than 400mg of vitamin E a day in the run-up to your surgery as it may interfere with blood clotting. Vitamin E is commonly included in multivitamins and antioxidant supplements, but check all labels and add up the dosages to ensure you do not exceed this limit. Just to be on the safe side, we would advise you to cut out any tablets including vitamin E in the week before your surgery.

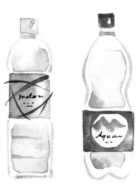

Your post-op supplement plan

After surgery we would recommend you continue with the pre-op plan for the next three months. You can also add in a few extras to help with healing:

1   Bromelain: an enzyme that has been shown to reduce tissue swelling and to increase the speed of healing. Take 500mg three times a day between meals and continue for seven to ten days after surgery.

2   Vitamin E oil can be applied topically to reduce scar formation (once the skin has closed over a healing wound).

Supplements to avoid

Certain supplements will interfere with the healing process. You will need to avoid the following for a month before surgery. NOTE: these are the most commonly used contraindicated supplements and do not constitute an entire list. You must tell your surgeon about *all* the medications, supplements and herbs you take at your consultation.

- Echinacea: can interfere with wound healing and may interact badly with drugs used during surgery.
- Ephedra (ma huang): can cause irregular heartbeat and problems with blood pressure and/or heart rate during surgery.
- Feverfew: may interfere with blood clotting and increase the risk of bleeding.
- Garlic: may increase the risk of bleeding.
- Ginger: may increase the risk of bleeding. NOTE: you can have ginger in food, it is just the high potency supplement form that is contraindicated.
- Gingko biloba: may increase the risk of bleeding.
- Ginseng (Panax ginseng): may increase the risk of clotting and interfere with anti-clotting drugs. It may increase heart beat and blood pressure under surgery.
- Goldenseal: may increase blood pressure and risk of swelling.
- Hypericum (St John's wort): may increase the effects of anaesthetic; may interfere with drugs used before, after and during surgery.
- Kava kava: may increase the effects of anaesthetic.
- Liquorice: may increase blood pressure; may create electrolyte imbalance.
- Omega-3 fish oils: may increase bleeding.
- Valerian: may increase the effects of anaesthetic.
- Vitamin E: may increase the risk of bleeding and affect clotting.

Homeopathic help

Homeopathy can prove invaluable in preparing the body for surgery and also helping it heal afterwards. Homeopathic remedies can be used safely in combination with surgery and there have been no reported problems in using them alongside cosmetic surgery. However, do please inform your surgeon that you are taking homeopathic remedies.

You might want to consider the following.

- Ferrum Phos (6x): four doses a day for two days prior to surgery is thought to help prevent infection.

- Arnica (30x): we always recommend our patients take Arnica. Ideally, take one dose the night before surgery; one in the morning on waking; one just before your surgery, one as soon after surgery as possible and another an hour after that. Then take as necessary until healing is complete.

- Gelsemium (30x): a useful remedy if you are very anxious or nervous about your surgery. Take one the night before surgery and one the morning of your surgery. If you are truly terrified of surgery (to the extent where you fear you might die) then substitute Aconitum 30x.

- Calendula and hypericum help to heal wounds and prevent infection. These can be applied topically; you can also buy a combined cream often called Hypercal.

- Apis can be helpful following procedures involving needles, such as Botulinum and fillers. Take 30x three times a day until symptoms are relieved.

- If you are having abdominal surgery, take Staphysagria 30x three times a day following surgery, until you feel better.

- If you are having breast surgery, take Bellis Perennis 30x three times a day following surgery, until you feel better.

- Homeopathic Anaesthetic (30x) should be taken three times a day following surgery to relieve the after-effects of anaesthetic.

- You can apply arnica cream or lotion following surgery on unbroken skin to help bruising and swelling. NOTE: do not use where the skin is broken.

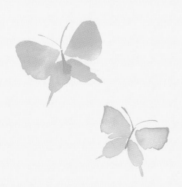

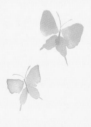

CHAPTER SEVEN

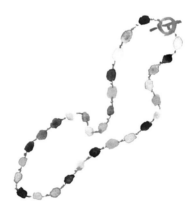

The lunchtime facelift:
non-invasive fixes

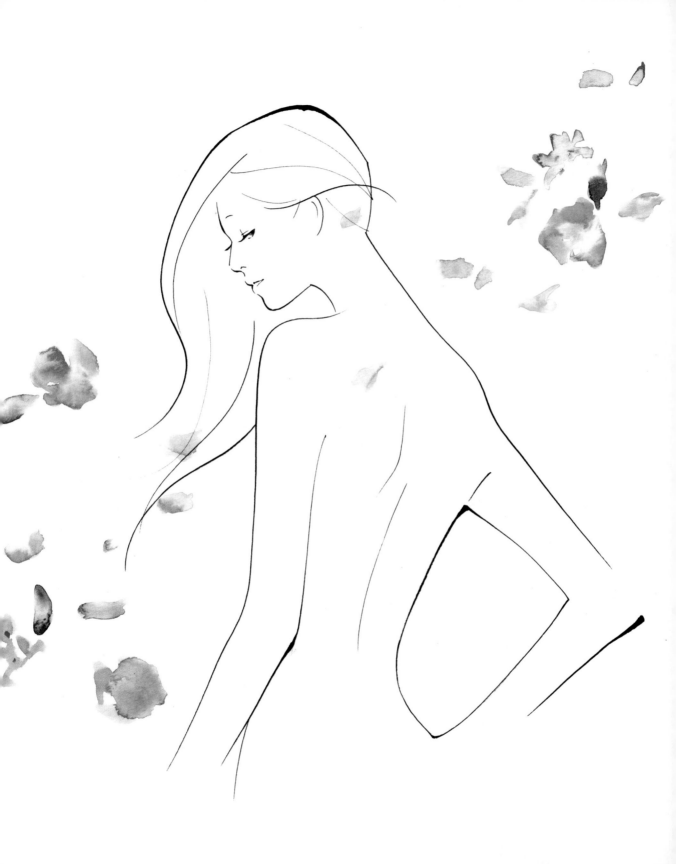

Welcome to the brave new world of cosmetic surgery. No knives, no general anaesthetics, no downtime. The papers have called it 'the lunchtime facelift' or 'lunchtime lipo' and, while not all these procedures are quite that swift, many really could fit into your lunch break. There are absolutely hordes of procedures that take from just ten minutes to about an hour – and that will make a heap of difference to how you look and feel. According to a survey in the *Economist*, a staggering 80 per cent of the increase in cosmetic surgery procedures is due to non-surgical procedures such as fillers, injections and peels. Last year British clinics carried out over 50,000 botulinum injections and around the same number of fillers were injected. Many surgeons believe that this is the future of cosmetic surgery and that we'll be swapping the scalpel for the syringe.

The benefits of non-invasive techniques are obvious. As you don't undergo extensive surgery (if indeed any surgery at all), there is less pain, less risk and much less recovery time required. Many people also like the fact that the results aren't always permanent – so if you change your mind or go off a look, you're not stuck with it (or with the need for corrective surgery).

Imagine it. You get up, look in the mirror and your mood instantly slumps. You're already looking tired (and you've only just woken up). Your skin appears grey and gaunt; there are crow's feet round your eyes and a permanent furrow in your forehead. You look much older than you really are and you go into work feeling rather low. Of course, you could just grimly grin and bear it but you decide to make a change. So, instead of having the usual lope around the shops at lunchtime, you get some botulinum injected. It takes the same amount of time and – hey presto – you no longer look like you're one of the cross brigade, about to launch into a tirade against the world. You're so pleased that you decide to go back next week to zap those crow's feet, and toy with the idea of a weekend peel to freshen up that city-stressed skin. Within a month your friends and colleagues are bemused. You look so much brighter, happier – younger.

So much modern cosmetic surgery is subtle, swift and non-invasive. Ten to one we now turn to the needle rather than the knife; we can peel and resurface the skin, rather than cutting and splicing it. Of course, botulinum is the best known of the new non-invasive techniques, but there are plenty of other options. In fact you'll be spoiled for choice. So this section of the book will tell you exactly what's what: what each of these new techniques does (and what it can't do); how long it lasts; and if you need to be wary of any side effects. Just because these techniques are non-invasive doesn't mean they are suitable for everyone – you need to choose your procedure with care.

NOTE: prices will vary enormously across the country and in individual clinics. We have, however, tried to give an indication of price, as follows:

- *Low: under £1,000 for the procedure or course of treatments*
- *Medium: up to £3,000*
- *High: £3,000 plus*

Your face

REVITALISING FACE TREATMENTS

Not everyone needs a full-on facelift. There are plenty of anti-ageing treatments that can tone, strengthen and rejuvenate facial skin. The mildest procedures are either totally non-invasive or minimally so, and either totally painless or merely involve a little discomfort. Techniques such as micro-currents, radio waves, pulsed light or facial acupuncture can brighten your face and minimise fine lines and wrinkles without even the sight of a scalpel. While a few offer pretty well instant results, don't expect sudden transformations with the majority of these techniques. Many require a course of treatment for the best results. Most will give you a subtle change, not a dramatic overhaul. Remember too that, while they will brighten your look and refine your skin tone, they may not be able to deal with deep-seated problems and advanced ageing. On the whole we would say they are primarily preventative treatments that may well dramatically reduce your need for more invasive treatment later on. They will also work wonders in conjunction with surgical procedures; we often recommend them before and after facelifts, brow lifts and so forth.

The following will all give an all-over lifting and rejuvenating effect to your face and won't require you to take time off work. Some, like CACI, will probably already be familiar names. But this is a field that is growing all the time and new advances come in swift and fast. Although the choice might seem excessive, it is actually a good thing. We need plenty of options so that we can tailor your treatment to your lifestyle. Some treatments are very expensive and it's good to be able to offer choices to suit most incomes. Equally, some treatments are very time-consuming and not everyone can give up the amount of time needed for a course of treatments so, again, with a large choice we can find something that will fit into your life. Then again, you might not like needles (however tiny) or be uneasy about the idea of micro-currents pulsing through your skin. Whatever your preference, there will be something to suit.

We've outlined the treatments you are most likely to come across, and we give you our honest appraisal of how good they really are.

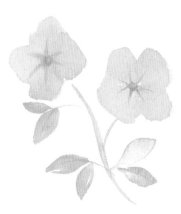

FACTFILE: MICRO-CURRENT

- Other names: CACI, non-surgical facelift.

- How does it work? Micro-currents of electricity stimulate muscles, leading to an increase in production of protein which, in turn, causes them to tighten and firm.

- What's it good for? Sun-damaged skin, fine lines and wrinkles, poor muscle tone, uneven pigmentation, acne scarring; tightening facial contours, improving circulation.

- What happens? Cotton-tipped probes and pads are placed on your face (or body) and the machine is turned on and adjusted to a comfortable level. Rhythmic pulses then go through your face or body.

- How does it feel? Rather like pins and needles; sometimes it feels as if your skin is being gently pulled and then released.

- How long does it take? A session takes about an hour (you will need a course of ten treatments ideally).

- How long before it heals? There is no damage to the skin so healing is instantaneous.

- When will I see results? Most people notice results after about four or five sessions.

- How long will it last? For optimum results you need monthly maintenance sessions.

- Any side effects? None is known. Micro-current started off as a medical treatment to help facial weakness in people with palsy. It has been extensively tested and is quite safe.

- Contraindications? None.

- Most suitable age to have it? Mid-thirties and over.

- Cost? Low.

We say: It's a perfectly decent, well-established treatment. The results aren't permanent, but with persistence they can be long-lasting.

FACTFILE: LIFT 6

- Other names: Cosmecanique.

- How does it work? It uses rhythmical pulsation to stimulate the connective tissue and the production of collagen in order to tone, strengthen and rejuvenate your facial skin. It is also a superb lymphatic drainage technique.

- What's it good for? Firming loose skin, crow's feet, wrinkles between the eyebrows and around the lips; making skin feel and look fresher and younger. The drainage effect can help puffiness enormously.

- What happens? All make-up is taken off and then a therapist moves the hand-held machine over your skin, depending on your individual needs: all over the face, neck and jawline; sometimes very gently and minimally around the eye area.

- How does it feel? It is totally painless and most people find it very soothing and relaxing.

- How long does it take? Sessions last for thirty minutes. A course of ten sessions is recommended, twice weekly, to achieve best results.

- How long before it heals? There is no downtime.

- When will I see results? You will notice a difference after one treatment but best results come after three or four sessions.

- How long will it last? To maintain results you will need top-up sessions once a month.

- Any side effects? No.

- Contraindications? Inflammation or infection of the skin; oedema; eczema/psoriasis; herpes; infected acne.

- Most suitable age to have it? Any age. It can target the first signs of ageing in younger women (twenties plus) and equally help mature skin (thirties plus).

- Cost? Low.

We say: This is a treatment we use in our clinic – and it gets great results. It offers a simple and effective workout that tones, strengthens and rejuvenates your facial skin. It also gives a gentle exfoliating effect, so that even after one session the skin will look and feel younger and softer.

CASE STUDY

Susan Carney is an accountant in her late twenties. She lives in Berkshire.

I suppose I'm a typical hard-working, hard-playing twenty-something. I don't eat the best possible diet, I do drink a bit more than I should and I don't get to the gym that often either. I spend a fortune on beauty treatments though and am often pretty dissatisfied with the results they give. Most of the beauty business is sheer hype. I've always been pretty happy with my face. I like what I see in the mirror on the whole. But when I saw some photos of me on holiday last year I was horrified. My face is fine from the front but my profile was awful. I was getting a double chin and my profile really lacked tone and definition. It was a bit of a wake-up call really.

I went to the Centre and saw Maurizio. I said I wanted a thread lift but he wouldn't countenance it. He said my skin simply didn't need it. He read me the riot act a bit on my diet and the booze. He also guilt-tripped me into getting a personal trainer. He said if I wanted a good toning effect I could have Lift 6. I was a bit sceptical to be truthful – it sounded like just another salon treatment. But I have to say I was proved wrong. I had the full course and it really made a difference, toning and firming up my face. It's also really enjoyable – you just lie back and enjoy it. It feels like a gentle suction all over your face – a strange feeling but really rather nice. I have to admit Maurizio was right, and now I'm really pleased I didn't have invasive surgery. I'm keeping up with a maintenance programme now and can face the camera with a lot more confidence.

FACTFILE: PERFECTOR

- How does it work? It uses a combination of electric currents (micro-current, frequency and waveform) to work deeply into the skin and muscle to increase metabolism, circulation and speed up cellular activity.

- What's it good for? Fine lines and wrinkles, cellulite; skin contouring and firming of sagging skin.

- What happens? Your skin is cleansed and toned. A micro-current gel is applied to the area being treated. The machine has two electrodes that deliver currents to the skin in various stages (stimulating circulation, encouraging lymphatic drainage, lifting and firming muscles).

- How does it feel? As if your skin is being massaged – it's not unpleasant.

- How long does it take? A session lasts around forty-five minutes.

- How long before it heals? There is no damage to the skin so no healing time is required.

- When will I see results? Often after the first session. For best results you should have a course of six to ten treatments.

- How long will it last? Follow-up treatments are recommended every six months to maintain results.

- Any side effects? None.

- Contraindications? None.

- Most suitable age to have it? Thirties and upwards.

- Cost? Low.

We say: It's another alternative, but again the benefits will only be temporary.

FACTFILE: THERMAGE

- Other names: Thermacool, Thermalift.

- How does it work? Radio frequencies warm the collagen in the dermis which tighten and thus lift and contour the skin. The top layers of the skin are left completely alone, hence there is no downtime.

- What's it good for? Fine lines and wrinkles, acne scarring, overly oily skin; skin contouring and firming of sagging skin.

- What happens? A local anaesthetic cream is often applied to minimise discomfort. A hand-held device sends the radio frequencies to the areas being treated.

- How does it feel? A little uncomfortable on the less fleshy areas of the face, but not painful.

- How long does it take? Sixty to ninety minutes.

- How long before it heals? There is no damage to the skin so no healing time is required.

- When will I see results? Often immediately, although the best effects appear after about two to six months, as new collagen is produced.

- How long will it last? Up to about five years. Some people will need top-up treatments before this time, depending on your skin.

- Any side effects? Your skin may be a little red for a few hours following treatment.

- Contraindications? Pregnancy. Breastfeeding. Pacemakers or metal implants in the face (excluding fillings). You would need to wait six months after Roaccutane treatment, chemical peels and dermal fillers.

- Most suitable age to have it? Mid-thirties and upwards.

- Cost? High.

We say: It's new and a good non-invasive treatment that will be very important in the future. It's going to be big.

FACTFILE: LIGHT THERAPY

- Other names: Lumiere, Omnilux Revive.

- How does it work? Pure red light from LEDs (light emitting diodes) is focused on the face; this emits the correct wavelength of light to stimulate collagen and elastin production.

- What's it good for? Spots, blemishes, uneven skin tone, fine lines and wrinkles, particularly forehead worry lines. Can also be therapeutic for sufferers of SAD (seasonal affective disorder, or the Winter Blues). Often used to prolong the effects of fillers and Botulinum toxin.

- What happens? The lamp is warmed up and then you simply lie down on a couch with the lamp positioned over your face. You relax until the machine automatically switches off.

- How does it feel? Very pleasant and warm, like lying on a sunbed.

- How long does it take? Twenty minutes.

- How long before it heals? Instantly.

- When will I see results? You should notice your skin appearing more vibrant after just one session, but full results come after six to twelve treatments.

- How long will it last? You will need monthly or bi-monthly top-ups to maintain results.

- Any side effects? Very unlikely.

- Contraindications? Light sensitivity or if you are on light sensitising medications or herbs.

- Most suitable age to have it? Any.

- Cost? Low.

We say: It is very pleasant, a very enjoyable feeling – it doesn't provide miracles but it gives you a definite feeling of well-being after the treatment.

FACTFILE: MESOLIFT

- Other names: Meso-Rejuv; Meso-Skin, Vita Facelift.

- How does it work? A blend of micronutrients is injected into the skin. These include vitamins, minerals, amino acids, co-enzymes and nucleic acids. They combine to help hydrate the skin, promote the natural production of collagen and elastin, and improve circulation, hence firming and toning the skin, and tautening facial contours.

- What's it good for? Fine lines and wrinkles; tightening face and neck.

- What happens? You may be given a local anaesthetic gel before injections with a tiny needle insert the nutrient mix into your face and neck.

- How does it feel? You may feel light pinpricks.

- How long does it take? Thirty minutes.

- How long before it heals? More or less immediately.

- When will I see results? Many people notice results after just one session, although generally a course of up to six treatments is recommended.

- How long will it last? The effects are cumulative, so it is recommended that you have twice-yearly top-ups to maintain results.

- Any side effects? This is a very safe treatment as the micronutrients are those found in the skin. Your skin will be a little red after the treatment but this will fade in a few hours. Your skin may feel tight for several days and there may be some light bruising.

- Contraindications? Pregnancy, breastfeeding, insulin-dependent diabetics; people with a history or high risk of stroke, blood clots; people with heart disease (on medication).

- Most suitable age to have it? All ages.

- Cost? Low.

We say: This is a good non-invasive alternative that gives deep nutrition to the skin. We are introducing a similar treatment at our own Centre – bioregeneration injections that can plump up the skin, improve collagen and lift the skin around the jaw, cheeks and the eyebrow area.

FACTFILE: SUPERFICIAL PEEL

- How does it work? A mild chemical solution (most likely glycolic or fruit peel) removes the outer layers of skin, working like a good exfoliating scrub.

- What's it good for? Uneven pigmentation, fine lines and wrinkles; freshening tired, jaded skin, mild skin damage (caused by sun/acne/scarring).

- What happens? The solution is applied to your face and left for a short period of time.

- How does it feel? It may feel a little warm or tight.

- How long does it take? About ten to fifteen minutes.

- How long before it heals? About two days (but you will be able to go back to work immediately, as any pinkness can be covered by light make-up).

- When will I see results? A few days.

- How long will it last? About four to six weeks (you will need top-ups monthly for best results).

- Any side effects? The skin will be a little pink to begin with. There is a very slight risk of infection, scarring or hyperpigmentation (treated areas turn overly pale).

- Contraindications? Peels are not suitable for people on acne drugs (Roaccutane, etc.) and steroids. They are not suitable for dark skin.

- Most suitable age to have it? Teens upwards.

- Cost? Low.

We say: This can be a good starting point for having skin treatments. It's an easy treatment that can give a real glow to your skin. It's very good for younger people, including teenagers. It can reduce sun damage.

FACTFILE: MICRODERMABRASION

- How does it work? It is similar to dermabrasion but uses very tiny crystals to 'sand down' the skin surface, and is far gentler and less intrusive. Polishes the surface of the skin and also stimulates circulation to help produce fresh healthy skin.

- What's it good for? Finer lines and wrinkles, sun damage, superficial scarring, very superficial acne scarring.

- What happens? A device like a fine sandblaster sprays tiny crystals across the face which, together with gentle abrasion, removes the dead outer layer of skin (but nowhere near as much depth of skin as dermabrasion).

- How does it feel? You feel a mild roughness, like a very stringent exfoliation.

- How long does it take? Around thirty-five minutes per treatment; you will need up to six treatments for the best effects.

- How long before it heals? Pretty much immediately.

- When will I see results? Skin often looks brighter and feels smoother after one session; best results are seen as sessions continue.

- How long will it last? You will need monthly touch-ups to maintain results.

- Any side effects? No, microdermabrasion is very gentle.

- Contraindications? None.

- Most suitable age to have it? Any.

- Cost? Low.

We say: This is a good maintenance treatment, a high street beauty treatment that helps to exfoliate and keep the skin clean.

WHAT ELSE IS THERE OUT THERE?

- **Oxygen therapy**: uses a combination of facials, creams and simply blasting the skin with oxygen to freshen and lighten skin. Regular treatment gives best results.

- **Rejuvanessence**: gentle yet effective facial massage that stimulates circulation and releases muscle tension to give a natural lift. You need a course of about ten sessions. Practitioners will usually do one side at a time, allowing you to see the difference halfway through the session.

- **Acupuncture**: facial acupuncture stimulates energy flow and releases muscle tension, diminishing lines, uneven skin tone, scars and dark circles. Three or more sessions are required. If you don't like needles, there are also acupressure-based treatments in which finger pressure is used to stimulate the required points.

- **Revitale**: a vitamin/mineral/amino acid/herbal compound is painted on to the skin where it dries like a mask. The active compounds are said to help the skin repair and rejuvenate. It tightens loose skin and can lessen wrinkles. You need about four treatments.

- **Beautytek**: a wonderful new energy treatment that gives a distinct lift to the face. We will talk about it in greater depth in the Body section of this chapter (see page 143). But do consider it as a very viable natural lifting, firming and freshening treatment for the face. We are very excited about it.

SPOT TREATMENTS FOR PROBLEM AREAS

There are also some good minimally invasive treatments for specific areas of the face. If you are bothered by spider veins or specific furrows or lines, these could be the treatments for you. Again, you will be able to go straight back to work and normal life following these treatments.

FACTFILE: MICROWAVE TREATMENT

- Other names: Veinwave, V-Beauty.

- How does it work? A high-frequency microwave heats and destroys thread veins (a process called thermocoagulation).

- What's it good for? Thread veins, rosacea.

- What happens? A very fine needle is inserted into the vein; a microwave is administered and the vein is reabsorbed into the body. The outer layers of skin are left undamaged.

- How does it feel? You can feel the warmth under the skin, which can be a little uncomfortable.

- How long does it take? Sessions last up to thirty minutes (during which around 50cm of veins can be treated). If you have large areas of problematic veins you will need several sessions.

- How long before it heals? Nearly instantaneously.

- When will I see results? It depends on the individual. Usually after a week to six weeks.

- How long will it last? Usually permanently.

- Any side effects? There may be some redness for up to six weeks. The procedure is very safe and scarring is extremely rare.

- Contraindications? Pregnancy. If you have a pacemaker or if you suffer from epilepsy.

- Most suitable age to have it? All ages.

- Cost? Low.

We say: This is a good treatment for thread veins. It's probably the easiest treatment available, and very safe.

FACTFILE: INTENSE PULSED LIGHT (IPL)

- Other names: Epilight, Vasculight, Multilight, PhotoFacial.

- How does it work? It's not a laser (which only uses one wavelength of light), but rather short pulses of broad-spectrum light are directed into the skin. This heats the lower levels of the skin causing mild damage, which stimulates the skin to produce collagen for repair. The epidermis is unharmed. The system filters the light carefully so the harmful shorter wavelengths are removed.

- What's it good for? Uneven pigmentation, melasma, rosacea, broken capillaries, age spots and sunspots. It is also frequently used for hair removal.

- What happens? Your skin is analysed. A local anaesthetic and then cold gel are applied to your face and the light is then pulsed at your face through a glass handpiece. A computer program ensures you will receive the right amount of treatment for your skin type.

- How does it feel? You may experience warmth and some mild stinging.

- How long does it take? About half an hour. It's usually advisable to have a series of between three and six sessions, about a month apart.

- How long before it heals? There is no downtime as the epidermis is unharmed.

- When will I see results? Usually after about two to three weeks.

- How long will it last? For optimum long-term results you will need top-ups every six months.

- Any side effects? Immediately after treatment, warmth, redness and tingling. Rare complications include blistering of the skin which can lead to changes in skin colour and/or slight scarring.

- Contraindications? Pregnancy. If you have used Roaccutane up to six months before treatment. You must avoid sunbeds or being in the sun for six weeks before treatment.

- Most suitable age to have it? Thirties upwards.

- Cost? Low to medium.

We say: It's a good treatment, a maintenance treatment to keep a good complexion and to follow up after more invasive therapies – no downtime, excellent and safe.

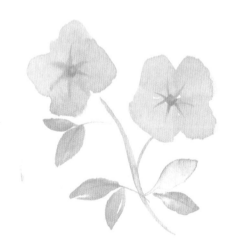

Botulinum: the modern miracle

Whatever did we do before Botox? Botulinum toxin is the most popular cosmetic procedure: over 100,000 injections are given in the UK every year. It's the perfect lunchtime procedure as it is so swift and requires no recovery time. Some women even have Botox parties, where they club together to hire a surgeon and sip champagne while having their frown lines ironed out. However, as much fun as it sounds, we would not advise this as it's never wise to mix cosmetic surgery (however non-invasive) with alcohol. Plus we would always recommend you have any procedure carried out in a clinic, rather than your own home, to ensure you are being treated by a skilled surgeon or dermatologist and to minimise any risk. It's highly unlikely that anything would go wrong, but better safe than sorry.

Let's clear up the name business before we go any further. Botox is simply a trade name used for botulinum toxin type A. Dysport is another (and happens to be the one we use). Another type of botulinum, type B (with the trade name Myobloc), is also used for cosmetic surgery. On the whole, cosmetic surgeons prefer type A because it is longer-lasting than type B and less expensive. Type B does act faster though, and can be used as an alternative if you build up antibodies against type A so it ceases to work. Just to confuse you further, the name Botox itself is no longer used for cosmetic work. In 2006 Botox became known under its new trade name Vistabel. To avoid any more confusion we'll stick to the generic botulinum from now on in this book!

Botulinum toxin comes from the bacterium **Clostridia botulinum**, an unpleasant creature that can cause the nasty illness botulism. Fortunately in its purified protein form it is totally safe and has, in fact, been used for many years for medical purposes. It made its first surgical appearance way back in 1822 when a German doctor found it could help people with excessive sweating (by blocking the sympathetic nerve fibres that control the sweat glands). It is still used for this very successfully, and is also used to correct squints, prevent spasms of the eyelids, and ease the symptoms of cerebral palsy.

Botulinum toxin is popular for very good reasons. It's a simple, straightforward, highly effective alternative to surgery for the elimination of fine lines. We use it a lot in our practice and our patients like it enormously (as does Maurizio). Facial lines, as we've seen, are frequently caused by the repeated use of the facial muscles in a certain way. While we can soften or even erase lines with filler injections or peels, botulinum treatment is different as it is a preventative treatment as well as a cure. Injections are given usually to the forehead area, temporarily putting the frown muscles to sleep for between three and six months. This freezing does not permanently affect the muscle, but just allows it to 'hibernate', if you like, for a few months. The idea is to break the habit of frowning and re-educate your facial movements, so you eventually forget how to frown. Result? No more lines.

Some people are concerned that they are being injected with a substance that derives from an unpleasant disease-causing organism. Don't be. Botulinum toxin cannot cause any permanent damage and it can't travel inside the body because it attaches itself firmly to the muscle and cannot move away from it. There is no risk of it passing into the bloodstream. Trust us.

FACTFILE: BOTULINUM TOXIN INJECTION

- Other names: Botox (Vistabel), Dysport, Myobloc.

- How does it work? Botulinum toxin is a purified protein that blocks the nerve signal from the brain to the nerve endings (that tell you to frown). Injecting botulinum into the skin effectively paralyses the muscles, so wrinkles, lines and furrows don't have the strength to contract and simply have to smooth out.

- What's it good for? Crow's feet, forehead lines, lines around the mouth, upper lip lines, neck wrinkles, deep lines in the face, dimpling on the chin, lines on the chest.

- What happens? Botulinum toxin is injected into the problematic areas using a very fine needle. You may require several injections, depending on the extent of the problem.

- How does it feel? You will feel pinpricks but it isn't really painful.

- How long does it take? From ten to twenty minutes.

- How long before it heals? Immediately. You can go straight back to your life.

- When will I see results? Between one and three days after treatment.

- How long will it last? Up to six months (though can be less). After this the benefits continue in a modified form, as wrinkles relax and lines may simply diminish. However, for best results, you should return for top-ups at regular intervals.

- Any side effects? Botulinum is very safe. In rare cases, redness, swelling, bruising and numbness may occur initially. Headaches may happen. Very rare side effects include drooping of the eyelid or eyebrow (ptosis), frozen face syndrome, where you can no longer use your face expressively (this usually occurs only if you have a lot of injections in different sites around your face); the wrong muscle could be paralysed (but remember, botulinum is not a permanent treatment so the effect would be temporary).

- Contraindications? Not suitable if you are pregnant or breastfeeding. Botulinum is not suitable for people taking muscle relaxants (see your surgeon). You should avoid other procedures (micro-current, laser treatment, microdermabrasion etc.) for a week after treatment.

- Most suitable age to have it? Thirties.

- Cost? Low.

We say: Why have lines when such a simple, effective procedure can get rid of them? This is a treatment I (Maurizio) use for my own forehead and I love the results.

Cosmetic surgeons are pioneering all kinds of additional uses for botulinum, some of them quite surprising. Watch out for:

- Botulinum for breasts: it can relax the muscles that pull the breasts down, so the opposing muscles take over and lift them up. But it will only work for smaller breasts that haven't drooped too far.

- Botulinum for calves: a shot of botulinum can shave a few millimetres off calf muscles – handy if you can't quite squeeze into your favourite boots.

- Botulinum for scar reduction: by relaxing the region around an operation site, botulinum can cause less pull and hence lessen the chance of wide or irregular scars.

- Botulinum for nose jobs: if your muscles are creating a downward pull, botulinum could help the shape of a droopy nose tip.

- Botulinum for a better smile: no, it can't fix your teeth but if the corners of your mouth are pulling down, giving you a gloomy look, it can help the muscles relax back to neutral. It can also prevent a gummy grin by narrowing your smile so it's just your teeth on show.

- Botulinum as facelift: by injecting botulinum into the cords of the neck, it's possible to give the lower face and mouth a slight lift and eliminate many lines in the neck. This requires a specialist surgeon as it's a tricky procedure.

- Botulinum as brow lift: injecting the muscles over the brows lifts up excess skin over the eyes, making eyes seem larger and more open.

   We say: While these are exciting developments, do bear in mind they are new applications. You would need to find a surgeon who is very experienced, not just in normal botulinum toxin injections, but specifically in these new areas.

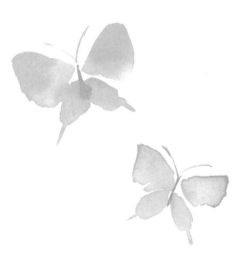

CASE STUDY

Eleanor Lindsay, fifty, is a nurse from Surrey.

I'm really lucky in that I'm blessed with great skin and people regularly think I'm twenty years younger than I am. I'm not remotely vain and had never considered cosmetic surgery – I'm much more of a natural treatment person really. I make sure I eat a great diet and I have regular massage. But, five years ago, when I saw the beginnings of a frown I thought, I can't be having that. I actually don't mind lines but I hated the fact that I looked permanently cross. I looked in the mirror and thought, I don't look how I feel, and that was horrible.

I don't look forward to the needles. You can feel it going in and it does hurt a bit, but it's nothing major – you're not passing out or anything. I simply go home, with maybe a tiny mark and then forget all about it. You notice the effect after a day or so. I have it done about twice a year, if that; the more I've had the less I've needed as your forehead forgets how to frown and so the lines automatically lessen. Roberto won't do it anyway unless he feels I really need it.

If you're thinking of botulinum I'd say catch it early, before the lines are really entrenched. By having it as a maintenance I know I won't get deep lines and will probably avoid needing fillers and other treatments later on.

One nice side effect is that it has slightly arched my eyebrows – it gives them a more defined, and much nicer, shape.

I'm not remotely a high-maintenance person but this is something I do to make me feel good. Basically it stops me worrying about looking worried!

THE GOOD FILLER GUIDE

It sounds rather like something you'd expect from a DIY shop, doesn't it? Well, actually, that's not so far from the truth. Just as you can plug gaps in your walls and woodwork with various fillers, so the creases and crevices of your face can be, shall we say, *smoothed* (plugged isn't a good word when applied to faces) with clever new dermal fillers and implants. These are, simply put, materials that we inject or insert into the skin wherever it needs to be plumped up or firmed. They can fill in wrinkles, lines, folds and furrows but can also give a youthful plumpness to saggy cheeks or thinning lips. They can give you 'cheekbones' or subtly alter the shape of your face.

These are very clever substances and often take away or delay the need for more invasive treatments. However they do have limits. If you have deep folds in the face or brow, caused by overactive muscles or loose skin, you may need a facelift or brow lift for the best effect. Equally, fillers are not usually sufficient to cope with severe surface wrinkles, such as multiple vertical 'lipstick' lines that can form around the mouth. In this case, one of the resurfacing methods we will discuss later would produce a smoother appearance and be the treatment of choice.

What's really exciting is the huge range of fillers and implants available. Some are strictly temporary, lasting only a few months, while others can last you for life. We often find that our patients like to try out an effect with a temporary filler. If they don't like it, it really doesn't matter as it simply won't last that long. However, if they love the look, they can then choose to repeat the temporary injections or opt for something lower maintenance and longer lasting. Equally, you have a wide choice when it comes to the kind of filler or implant you use: synthetic or natural, animal-based or not, beads or gels.

You can even use your own fat cells, something that many women find appealing – you are simply using your own fat, not some foreign substance. This procedure, which we are using more and more, is known as Fat Transplant or Lipofixing. Your own fat is harvested from somewhere like your abdomen, purified and then injected back into your face or wherever needs a boost. It's a totally natural and highly effective treatment. It's also possible to freeze harvested cells so they can be used for future touch-ups. It's very safe as there is no chance of allergic reactions because you are simply injecting your own cells back – just into a different bit of the body! However, it's worth pointing out that this is a slightly more invasive technique and will involve some bruising and swelling, plus the odd stitch.

Another development is even more subtle. Autologous Cell Therapy (ACT, often known as Isolagen) actually grows your own filler from a sample of your skin cells before it is injected back into your face (or other parts of the body). Brave New World indeed. This treatment also gives your collagen a bit of a kick up the backside, stimulating cell production and hence promising a huge improvement in skin tone, texture and elasticity, smoothing wrinkles and soothing scars. As with Fat Transplant, the appealing plus point for many women is that it's all totally natural. However it's still early days with this treatment and we have found that the results are not always predictable.

With such a huge choice, you will definitely need the guidance of a good cosmetic surgeon before making your final decision. However it's useful to get a broad idea of what's out there, so here are the factfiles.

FACTFILE: TEMPORARY FILLERS

- How do they work? The filler is injected into the area that needs filling or plumping, literally plumping out the line or area.

- What are they good for? Crow's feet, forehead lines, lines around the mouth, smile lines, nose to mouth lines (nasolabial creases), skin depressions and some scars; smoothing chin and cheek contours, smoothing wrinkles on the hands; increasing the volume of the lips.

- What happens? A local anaesthetic is given. A fine needle injects the filling material along or around the area to be treated. Different products are injected into different layers of the skin.

- How does it feel? It depends how the anaesthetic is applied; with a good anaesthetic, you should not feel any pain either during or after the procedure. However, if not, you could experience a certain amount of burning or stinging.

- How long does it take? Very much depends on the filler – around half an hour.

- How long before it heals? There is no downtime as such but you may feel numb for a few hours following treatment because of the local anaesthetic used.

- When will I see results? Immediately, but for best results once swelling disappears after one or two days.

- How long will it last? Between six months and two years (for best results you will need repeat injections, again from six-monthly to every two years).

- Any side effects? There may be some initial swelling and bruising. If you are having bovine collagen fillers you will need an allergy test, as up to 4 per cent of people are allergic to it. Complications are infrequent but can include infection, allergic reaction, abscesses, open sores, skin peeling, bruising, scarring and lumpiness.

- Contraindications? Pregnancy. An allergy to a particular filler (usually the bovine variety). Bovine collagen is contraindicated if you suffer from any of the following: auto-immune conditions, specifically rheumatoid arthritis; psoriatic arthritis; polymyositis; discoid lupus erythematosus. People with cold sores will need to be treated with extreme care (and with the use of antiviral medication).

- Most suitable age to have it? Thirties and forties.

- Cost? Low to medium (depending on filler used).

We say: A very effective, safe treatment. We particularly like Hydra Fill, a new biodegradable hyaluronic acid-based implant that is injected directly into the skin to restore or preserve a youthful-looking appearance. It is particularly effective for reducing nose-to-mouth grooves, frown lines and other depressed scars. It's also a godsend for enhancing narrow lips, and may even be used in the delicate tissue around the eyes. We use it because we have found it gives the best results and does not usually require an allergy test.

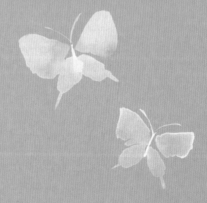

Types of temporary filler

These are the most common temporary fillers you will be offered. Surgeons all have their particular favourites. Collagen used to be very common, but increasingly surgeons (us included) are using hyaluronic acid because the results are so good. But really it's totally up to you. It very much depends on whether you have a preference for a natural substance or synthetic and how long you want the results to last.

- **Bovine-based collagen** (Zyderm, Zyplast): derived from purified collagen harvested from cow hide. Used for wrinkles, lines and enhancing lips. The downside to bovine collagen is that up to 4 per cent of the population are allergic to it, so you will have to have a skin test four weeks prior to treatment. The effects last about six months.

- **Calcium Hydroxylapatite** (Radiance): a synthetic filler that mimics a substance found in bone. It is also used in dentistry. The body accepts the implant and, because it is porous, normal tissue integrates itself through it. Commonly used to add volume around the lips and eyes but can also be used to correct cheeks, chins, jawline and browbone. It comes in either a solid form or an injectable or spreadable paste.

- **Human-based collagen** (CosmoDerm, CosmoPlast, Dermalogen, Cymetra): usually used around the eyes and lips, and between the nose and lips. It lasts up to six months. It's popular because, as a substance found in the body, there is no risk of allergic reaction.

- **Hyaluronic acid** (Hydra Fill, Restylane, Perlane, Hylaform, Juvederm, Rofilan, AcHyal): a polysaccharide (a natural form of sugar) that exists in the body where its most important role is carrying water, providing volume and flexibility to the skin. It also has a vital role in cell growth. Various forms are used for different effects: finer forms can reduce wrinkles and lines, while others can be used for augmenting lips and sculpting the contours of the face. Effects last from four to twelve months. There are two basic types of hyaluronic acid. First is a genetically engineered (non-animal) form (such as Restylane, Perlane and Hydra Fill). Second there is an animal-derived form which comes from the combs of cockerels (such as Hylaform).

- **Polylactic acid** (Sculptra): a synthetic filler that is used more for sculpting larger areas than just filling wrinkles. A new long-lasting product that has proved to be very effective, in particular for people who are HIV positive. Its results are longer-lasting than many temporary fillers – usually about two years.

Permanent and semi-permanent fillers/implants

While temporary fillers are useful for trying out a look, if you want long-lasting results you might want to look at the new range of fillers and implants that offer permanent or, at the least, very long-lasting results. Be absolutely certain though that you have got exactly the look you want. Some implants can be removed but you might incur some scarring (and, of course, it does involve a further operation and cost).

Many surgeons champion a range of synthetic implants. On the whole they are well tolerated and accepted by the body, and in most cases the surrounding blood vessels and tissue simply grow through the implant. In this section we list the most common types and give a factfile on them.

We would point out that our own personal (and strong) feeling is that permanent synthetic implants are not the best or safest option. We do not use them in our practice at all. Let us explain our reasons.

- First, not all types have undergone rigorous testing. You must check the safety record and test criteria with your surgeon. They are more likely to cause allergic reactions.

- Second, we simply don't know the long-term effects and what reactions will happen down the line. They therefore limit the use of other fillers because of the possibility of cross-reactions with them.

- Third, what happens when you age, when the rest of your face starts to sag but you already have a permanent filler in place? It limits your options for future work. We always tell our patients that they must think of the future. Permanent fillers may seem like a quick, easy option but a quick fix is not always the best.

FACTFILE: SYNTHETIC FILLERS

- How do they work? Synthetic fillers or implants are injected or inserted to plump out the problem area.

- What are they good for? Lines around the eyes, sunken cheeks, lines between the nose and mouth (nasolabial creases), forehead wrinkles, skin furrows or depressions, weak chins; lip enhancement, nose remodelling, jawline, cheekbone and brow definition.

- What happens? The site is prepared with an antiseptic solution. Then local anaesthetic is used to numb the area to be treated. A small incision is made and tissue is gently lifted to create a small tunnel or pocket for the implant. The implant material is inserted and, if necessary, trimmed to fit before being sutured into position. Stitches are removed after five to seven days. Some fillers can be injected into position.

- How does it feel? Expect some soreness and discomfort afterwards, also some bruising and swelling.

- How long does it take? It depends on what's being done – usually around an hour.

- How long before it heals? From several days to a few weeks, depending on the filler and the size of the area being treated. You will need to stay indoors, out of the sun, until the redness and bruising disappears.

- When will I see results? Usually after the swelling subsides (about a week).

- How long will it last? It depends on how much filler is used and how deeply it is injected or inserted. It can last for several years or for the rest of your life. However it may be necessary to do top-ups to maintain the desired effect.

- Any side effects? Swelling, bruising, redness. Scarring, though this is usually minimal. Allergic reactions or hypersensitivity are possible with this kind of filler. Other side effects include infection, nerve damage, numbness, skin discolouration, hardness over the injected area, scarring of the injected area.

- Contraindications? Allergy or sensitivity to the filler used. Pregnancy or breastfeeding. Any auto-immune disease or poor immune function. Susceptibility to keloids. Steroid treatment.

- Most suitable age to have it? Forties upwards.

- Cost? Medium.

We say: Obviously it is your decision but we would strongly urge against the use of synthetic permanent fillers for the reasons already given.

Synthetic fillers have astoundingly complex chemical names – real tongue-twisters. Here's the low-down on what all those 'polys' mean.

- **Polyacrylamine** (Hydrophilic polyacrylamide, HPG, Aquamid, Argiform, DermaLive, Outline, Evolution): this is an implant made almost entirely from water (95–97 per cent), combined with a synthetic polymer to form a kind of silicone gel, very similar to the material used in soft contact lenses. This implant stays soft once injected, the water content being absorbed by the body while the soft, pliable HPG becomes encapsulated by natural tissue. It is used all over the face, for lines, wrinkles, filling lips and cheeks.

- **Polyethylene** (HDPE, Medpor, Prolene, Marlex): this is a porous synthetic polymer that is non-biodegradable and biologically inert. It is non-toxic and usually well tolerated by the body; because it is porous, it allows for soft tissue and vascular growth through it, helping to keep the implant in place. Usually used for chin and cheek implants.

- **Polymethyl-methacrylate** (PMMA, Artecoll, Artefill): this is made from tiny plastic beads (microspheres) mixed with another agent, usually hyaluronic acid or bovine collagen. The mix is injected underneath the skin and the beads become caught in a web of scar tissue. Obviously, if bovine collagen is used, you will need an allergy skin test before this treatment. It is used all over the face, for lines, wrinkles, filling lips and cheeks.

- **Polytetrafluorethylene** (PTFE, Gore-Tex, Gore SAM, SoftForm): you'll be more familiar with this under one of its trade names, Goretex, a highly versatile synthetic polymer based on carbon and fluorine. It's softer than silicone and more readily accepted by the body (it's used a lot in standard medical surgical procedures, as well as in waterproof clothing!); blood vessels will flow directly into and through it. It is used all over the face, for lines, wrinkles, filling lips and cheeks.

- **Polyalkylinide** (Bioalcamide): a product comprising 96 per cent water, and 4 per cent polymer. Used for volume replacement and filling lines.

- **Silicone** (dimethylsiloxane): this is solid silicone, quite different from the liquid-filled silicone used in breast implants. Solid silicone does not leach into the body and has been used since the 1950s in facial cosmetic surgery and in general surgical procedures (heart valve replacement, prostheses, etc.). It is manufactured in various degrees of hardness, and in fluid, gel and rubber forms. It is usually used on cheeks, chin, jawline and nose. In the USA injectable silicone (made from silicone oil) has now been approved by the FDA and is being used for lines, furrows and acne scarring.

There *is* a permanent natural solution that we like very much and one Maurizio uses himself: Fat Transplant, or Lipofixing. This is a more invasive technique than that required for temporary fillers such as Hydra Fill, but the results are excellent.

FACTFILE: FAT TRANSPLANT

- Other names: Lipofixing, Lipotransfer, Fat harvesting.

- How does it work? Fat is removed from a part of your body with abundant fat deposits, purified and then injected back into the part of your face or body that needs filling or contouring.

- What's it good for? Lines around the eyes, sunken cheeks, lines between the nose and mouth (nasolabial creases), forehead wrinkles, skin furrows or depressions; plumping out hands. By placing fat in the upper third of the face you get an uplift effect.

- What happens? You are either sedated or local anaesthetic is used. The harvesting area is chosen (usually the abdomen but fat can also be harvested from the thighs or hips). Fat is suctioned using a blunt 2–3 mm cannula (a liposuction tubular-shaped tool). The fat is then cleaned and filtered. The area of your face requiring rejuvenation is anaesthetised and the fat is very carefully and precisely injected back into your face. The amount of fat put into each area is always more than is needed as about 40–50 per cent will be absorbed by the body. We keep additional fat in the freezer for potential future sessions.

- How does it feel? You don't feel anything as you are sedated. Afterwards there may be some bruising, swelling and some slight discomfort.

- How long does it take? One hour plus.

- How long before it heals? You have to stay for up to two hours following surgery (if you have had sedation) and you will need painkillers and antibiotics. You will have to keep a compression bandage on the harvest area for a week and there will be a suture (stitch) that is removed after one week.

- When will I see results? Immediately following surgery. But best results when any swelling and bruising subsides (about a week).

- How long will it last? Most patients need around two to three sessions. Then the result is permanent.

- Any side effects? You should expect swelling or bruising for a few days (sometimes a few weeks). You will need to stay indoors, out of the sun, until the redness and bruising disappear. Scarring, but it's minimal. Lumps and bumps are possible. There is no fear of allergic reaction as the procedure uses your own tissue. If you put on weight, the injected area can become enlarged.

- Contraindications? Pregnancy, hyperthyroidism, too little body fat on the body.

- Most suitable age to have it? Most suitable for younger women in their thirties and forties.

- Cost? Medium.

We say: What's not to like about this treatment? It has huge benefits and very few downsides. It offers a great result, is permanent yet totally natural. Maurizio is very happy with his experience of it.

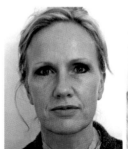 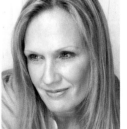

Before   *After*

CASE STUDY

Susannah Green, fifty-seven, is an office manager from Yorkshire.

They say your hands will always tell your age and I'd started becoming very aware that my hands were really giving mine away. The veins were looking more prominent and the skin was getting very thin. Cosmetic surgery hadn't crossed my mind – I wasn't for or against it, I had just never considered it could do anything for me.

Then I happened to be watching *Richard & Judy* one morning and there was a feature about hands: some women were trying very expensive hand creams while one had fat transplanted by Maurizio and Roberto. The fat transplant was really impressive – it beat the others hands-down, so to speak. I liked the fact that it was natural and relatively non-invasive so I decided to have it done for myself.

They took the fat from my abdomen under local anaesthetic. I was awake throughout, which I liked, and you really don't feel a thing – maybe just a little twinge. They took out more fat than was needed so they could freeze 5 litres in case I needed it later on (which seems such a sensible idea). There was a little swelling, because I do bruise easily but it goes down after a day or two and it's exciting because you notice the effects immediately.

I had my hands filled and also the lines from my nose to mouth, which had become quite pronounced. I had one treatment, then came back a month later for a follow-up. I was thrilled with the result. It's so natural yet the difference is really noticeable: my skin is really plumped up and the wrinkles just vanished.

I think it's a great treatment. It is quite expensive but I think it's worth every penny.

FACTFILE: AUTOLOGOUS CELL THERAPY (ACT)

- Other names: Isolagen.

- How does it work? A sample of your own cells is taken, cultivated in a laboratory and then injected back into your skin to boost your face's own production of healthy collagen and elastin.

- What's it good for? Crow's feet, forehead lines, lines from the nose to the mouth (nasolabial creases), wrinkles and fine lines on the face, acne scarring, lines and creases on the décolleté; plumping up hands.

- What happens? You are given a local anaesthetic and then a tiny incision is made behind your ear so a biopsy (skin sample) can be taken. This is then sent off to a laboratory where fibroblasts (collagen-producing cells) are grown. You return to your surgeon after about eight to ten weeks and the new cells are then injected into your face or elsewhere in the body.

- How does it feel? It is quite a painful treatment – you need ice, good topical cream and if you have a low pain threshold you should ask for sedation.

- How long does it take? A session lasts about thirty to forty-five minutes and you are advised to have two treatments, with a thirty to forty-five day interval between the two visits. The whole process takes about three months.

- How long before it heals? Skin heals swiftly after the biopsy as the sample is so small. The injections are very non-invasive and superficial and you should feel absolutely fine the day following surgery.

- When will I see results? It's a subtle treatment, results usually showing three to six months post-treatment. The increased fibroblast cells injected into your skin will continue to stimulate collagen and elastin production for around a year to eighteen months.

- How long will it last? Upwards of eighteen months. Yearly 'top-up' treatments are advised.

- Any side effects? Because ACT uses your own tissue, there is less risk of allergic reactions (though it is still possible). You will feel a little sore and have some reddening of the skin around the injection sites. There may be light bruising.

- Contraindications? ACT is not suitable during pregnancy. It should be avoided by women with auto-immune conditions and keloid scarring.

- Most suitable age to have it? Generally thirties to fifties. Some women in their twenties have collagen-producing cells stored ready for treatment in later life, or use the treatment for acne scarring.

- Cost? High.

We say: It is not a totally reliable treatment at the moment and there are a lot of potential pitfalls. Some people are very happy with the results while others don't see a big difference. It is a very expensive treatment and the (often small) result does not justify the cost in our opinion. Its best use is for acne scarring. Also, it's an option if you are nervous of other procedures. We do think it will improve in the future, however. Our advice? Best to wait for this one.

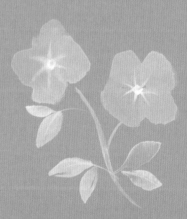

Your body

It's a sad fact of life that, as we get older, our bodies tend to sag more and more. There's a cruel irony in that fat disappears from the areas where you wish it wouldn't (your face, neck, hands) and starts to cluster in exactly the areas where you wish it wouldn't (bottom, hips, stomach, thighs). While excess weight is a nuisance, cellulite is the bugbear of virtually every woman out of her teens – nearly 80 per cent of women believe they suffer from it. Even if you don't suffer from cellulite you will probably feel unsatisfied with your skin tone and definition as you get older: buttocks and breasts seem less pert, while tummies and thighs seem to spread like butter on a warm day. Thread and spider veins can become obtrusive too, making you feel less confident about baring your body or wearing a bikini or shorts. While the obvious answer is for full-on cosmetic procedures, we also have a small armoury of non-invasive and less invasive techniques that can have surprisingly impressive effects.

LIPOSUCTION WITHOUT SURGERY?

Sometimes, no matter how much you diet, no matter how hard you exercise, there are bits of flab that just refuse to give up the ghost. Usually we turn to forms of liposuction, which we'll talk about later on. However sometimes that isn't totally necessary. If you have only minimal sagging or drooping, other less invasive techniques might do the trick. Liposuction without surgery? Is it really possible? Well, yes, to a degree. Don't expect these treatments to get rid of large areas of fat. They are not suitable if you are very overweight, so you would need to lose excess pounds first. Also they take a certain amount of persistence and commitment – they are not quick fixes by any means.

We use Endermologie a lot in our practice. It's an effective non-surgical treatment that reduces fat volume. Endermologie was originally developed in France where it was used in the treatment of burns, preventing skin from contracting and loosening scar tissue. The doctors using it noticed an interesting side effect: it improved the appearance of cellulite. This is one of the most widely approved treatments in the menu of cosmetic surgery, used in seventy countries by over 50,000 women every day. It has even been given approval by the American Food and Drug Administration (FDA). Other treatments are also excellent. We are increasingly impressed by Beautytek, and our colleagues report good results with a range of other treatments. We'll outline the most common and effective.

FACTFILE: ENDERMOLOGIE

- Other names: LPG, Liponic Sculpting.

- How does it work? It stimulates the superficial circulation of the body and the lymphatic circulation as well. It weakens the fibrous tissue and so minimises dimples and the appearance of cellulite. It can also stimulate the growth of collagen and elastin. This is a purely mechanical treatment using a suction and stretching movement with the aim of stretching the connective tissue.

- What's it good for? Cellulite, stubborn fat deposits, reducing fat volume. It is also highly effective when used in tandem with LipoSelection.

- What happens? You put on a body stocking and lie down on a couch. The therapist then uses a hand-held device that delivers constant or intermittent suction (depending on the programme being used) and rolling to the area being treated (and also the soft tissue below).

- How does it feel? It is painless and many patients even find the treatment soothing and relaxing. It's rather like a firm massage but with consistent pressure.

- How long does it take? Sessions last forty-five minutes. You will need to have twice-weekly treatments for a course of fourteen treatments.

- How long before it heals? There is no healing time.

- When will I see results? Fat break-up begins immediately so your body can look worse before the refining process takes place, usually around the fourth or fifth treatment.

- How long will it last? For best results we suggest a maintenance schedule of one treatment a month.

- Any side effects? It has been extensively studied and deemed to be very safe. It has FDA approval as an anti-cellulite treatment.

- Contraindications? Same as for any massage: infected or inflamed skin. Also high blood pressure.

- Most suitable age to have it? Any age. It is also very effective when used in combination with LipoSelection (used before and after surgery it shortens the recovery period by 50 per cent).

- Cost? Low.

We say: A very safe, well-researched treatment. To date no method has been found reliably and consistently to reduce the appearance of cellulite, but this is one of the best we have found.

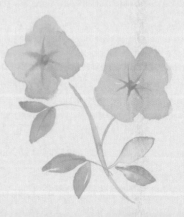

CASE STUDY

Susanna Mackie, thirty-eight, is a solicitor from London.

I'm a sporty person and I've always kept in good shape. I go to the gym regularly, I do ballet classes and I ski whenever I can. I'm pretty happy with my body on the whole but over the last year or so have really noticed cellulite building up on my thighs, the backs of my legs and on my abdomen. It's really horrible and, despite trying every cream, lotion and wrap going, nothing touches it.

I toyed with the idea of liposuction but wasn't quite ready for something that extreme. Then I heard about Endermologie and thought it was worth a go.

They put you in this skintight white suit made out of what looks like the same material as your tights – it's not a good look and I would have died if anyone other than the therapist had seen me! Then you lie down on the couch and the therapist starts working on you with this machine. It feels gorgeous – like a really strong sports massage. Your skin is lifted and kneaded all over and, though it is strong, it's also incredibly relaxing.

For the first few sessions I didn't notice any effects really – if anything it seemed to get worse. But I'd been told that could happen so I was expecting it. Apparently it's because the lymphatic system is geared up and your body is throwing off toxins. I drank lots of water to help the process and tried to eat well too. But after about the fourth session I really started noticing a difference. My skin started looking much smoother and it seemed to glow somehow. I definitely toned up too: I don't really weigh or measure myself but I noticed my trousers were looser on the legs. By the end of the course I had noticed a real difference. I didn't feel as if I needed to lurk in a corner of the changing room at my ballet class any more.

Now I go back for a top-up once a month – it's become part of my routine and I really love it. I'd say it's a brilliant treatment. In fact I bore for Britain about it to all my friends.

FACTFILE: ULTRASHAPE

- How does it work? High-frequency ultrasound is used to break down fat cells, which are then reabsorbed into the body.

- What's it good for? Stubborn areas of fat (particularly saddle-bags, love handles and flabby stomachs).

- What happens? You lie down and a handset is moved over the area being treated.

- How does it feel? A strange sensation, as if you are being injected but without any pinpricks. You may also feel warm and slightly uncomfortable.

- How long does it take? It depends on how many areas you have done, usually forty-five to ninety minutes. Most people have around three or four treatments.

- How long before it heals? There is no healing time. However you will be required to keep on a low-fat, low-carb diet for five days after each treatment to discourage the liquefied fat from relocating.

- When will I see results? Usually after two or more treatments.

- How long will it last? Results should be long-lasting, providing you do not put on weight.

- Any side effects? A few people experience bruising, but it's mild. Blistering is another very rare side effect.

- Contraindications? Pregnancy, breastfeeding, having a pacemaker, a history of blood coagulation disorder, abdominal hernia, metabolic disease.

- Most suitable age to have it? Any age.

- Cost? Medium.

We say: It can be very effective on small areas of fatty deposits, but it's a time-consuming treatment and expensive. It doesn't work so well for large areas or for general cellulite.

FACTFILE: VELASMOOTH

- How does it work? It uses radio waves, infrared light and vacuum suction to break down fatty deposits under the skin. Collagen growth is also stimulated to improve the skin from the inside out.

- What's it good for? Cellulite and stubborn fat deposits, particularly on the thighs and buttocks.

- What happens? The Velasmooth machine (which looks rather like an iron) rolls over the skin, pinching it upwards.

- How does it feel? As if you're being pinched or squeezed. You will also feel some warmth and tingling.

- How long does it take? A session lasts thirty to forty-five minutes and a course of twelve to sixteen is recommended.

- How long before it heals? There is no healing time. You will need to drink at least 2 litres of water during treatment as the lymphatic system is stimulated.

- When will I see results? Probably after about four or five sessions.

- How long will it last? Results should be long-lasting providing you do not gain weight.

- Any side effects? Redness and mild bruising, but this is rare. Blistering or burning is very rare but a faint possibility.

- Contraindications? Pregnancy, scarring, infection, having a pacemaker, diabetes, photosensitivity, thromboembolic conditions, taking anticoagulants.

- Most suitable age to have it? Any age.

- Cost? Medium.

We say: Many people like this; its effects are similar to those of Endermologie, but it also includes infrared light.

FACTFILE: BEAUTYTEK

- How does it work? Low-frequency electrical impulses are passed through the body encouraging fat to be broken down and collagen to grow.

- What's it good for? Cellulite, water retention, stretch marks. Mostly used on stomach, thighs, buttocks to reduce fat and is very effective at lifting small breasts. Also highly effective on the face where it gives a lifting effect.

- What happens? An electrolyte gel is applied to the area being treated, then a hand-held probe is passed over the area. You also hold a conductor so the machine can measure your responses and give the correct electrical stimulus needed for your individual body.

- How does it feel? Most people notice a tingle but a few people do find it slightly uncomfortable.

- How long does it take? Sessions last about an hour and you usually require a course of twelve (with two treatments per week).

- How long before it heals? No healing time.

- When will I see results? Usually you notice a difference after about two or three treatments.

- How long will it last? You will need to have maintenance treatments every three or four months to keep the effects.

- Any side effects? You may need to go to the toilet during or directly following treatment.

- Contraindications? Not suitable for women who are pregnant or breastfeeding; those with large metal implants (such as hip replacements), pacemakers, epilepsy or cancer.

- Most suitable age to have it? Any.

- Cost? Medium.

We say: It's a great new development and we're very excited about it. It gives a marked improvement in the appearance of cellulite and fat, but is totally non-invasive and safe. It can also be used very successfully on the face as a mild lift. We recommend it highly.

FACTFILE: MESOTHERAPY

- How does it work? By injecting hyaluronic acid into the skin to plump up and smooth the appearance of cellulite, and improve skin tone.

- What's it good for? Cellulite, poor skin tone, dry dehydrated skin. Most often used on the thighs, buttocks, back and stomach. It works well for people who are slightly overweight, but it can't treat loose or hanging skin.

- What happens? Small amounts of hyaluronic acid are injected into the skin.

- How does it feel? You will feel pinpricks but the needles are incredibly fine so, while it may be uncomfortable, it's not painful.

- How long does it take? It depends on the area being treated, usually between ten and thirty minutes. Between five to ten treatments are generally recommended.

- How long before it heals? Usually about one or two days.

- When will I see results? Gradually, over the course of treatment.

- How long will it last? You will need treatments every four to six months.

- Any side effects? Expect some redness, swelling, itching and tenderness for a few days. Small bruises may appear. Some people are hypersensitive to hyaluronic acid (it's very rare – about 1 in 10,000 people treated – and reactions last for only a week or so).

- Contraindications? Pregnancy, cancer, heart disease.

- Most suitable age to have it? Any.

- Cost? Medium.

We say: It's an older method developed in France and Italy. It can be a good option for skin rejuvenation on the face and décolleté. However, when it comes to fat reduction, we think the results are very limited as it will only tackle small localised fat deposits. Also the swelling, redness and itching may prolong the healing process. Consider carefully if it is really worth it.

OTHER OPTIONS

- **Thermage**: we discussed Thermage in the Face section. It uses radio frequencies to lift skin and its underlying tissues. Now it has been sanctioned for use as a body treatment, where it can firm up sagging stomachs, bottoms and thighs and tone flappy under-arms. Again, definitely one to watch. It will be an important treatment of the future.

- **TriActive**: combines laser treatment with massage to stimulate circulation and break down fat. It requires about twelve or fourteen one-hour sessions to get results. Anecdotal reports suggest results can be a little patchy but it works well for some people, giving a lifting, firming effect.

- **Manual Lymphatic Drainage (MLD)**: a very gentle form of massage that encourages lymphatic drainage. For such a minimal treatment it has surprisingly good results. For best results you learn how to massage yourself and use DIY treatments on a daily basis. It's superb for water retention, puffiness and reducing scars and stretch marks but it's time-consuming and you have to be willing to put in the work yourself.

- **Ionithermie**: a well-known hip and thigh smoothing beauty treatment that also helps reduce cellulite. It combines electric current therapy with thermal clay and algae masks. It requires around five treatments and is ideal for people who have lost weight but now want to firm up.

- **Micro-current treatment**: as discussed in the Face section. While most usually used for tightening up facial tissue, it can also help with body toning and poor circulation. Takes time and commitment and, to our mind, there are now more effective treatments. However the cost is low and so it's a good option if funds are tight.

LIPOSTABIL: A NOTE OF CAUTION

Lipostabil (also known as Lipodissolve, Flabjab, Fat-Away and Lipo-Melt) has been promoted as an alternative to liposuction. Its active ingredient is phosphatidylcholine, designed for the prevention and treatment of fat blockages in blood vessels. It has not been tested for safety as a cosmetic procedure and its manufacturers actively say it should not be injected subcutaneously (under the skin). Therefore the MHRA (the Medicines and Healthcare products Regulatory Agency, part of the Department of Health) does not approve its use and has issued warnings that it should not be used in cosmetic surgery. It is unlikely you will find this treatment in the UK but we feel it's important to point out the facts. There have been adverse reactions to this treatment when used cosmetically; while the idea of a 'flab jab' is intensely appealing, in practice it is not a viable or safe option as yet.

REMOVING THREAD/SPIDER VEINS

As if cellulite weren't enough, many women (particularly those who have had children) find they develop unsightly spider or thread veins, usually on the legs. These can now be removed simply using either microwave or IPL treatment (as discussed in the Face section), or sclerotherapy. Microwave and IPL are used for very fine veins (usually on the feet), while sclerotherapy takes care of slightly larger veins (but still very fine – showing up red). Do note that these treatments will not be suitable if you have varicose veins (larger, deeper, blue veins), in which case you will need to consult your doctor.

FACTFILE: SCLEROTHERAPY

- How does it work? Removes very fine veins by injecting them with a solution of sterile salt and anaesthetic that irritates and breaks down the walls of the vein. The collapsed vein disperses naturally through the body.

- What's it good for? Thread veins on the calves and thighs, spider veins, rosacea, port wine stains.

- What happens? The problematic vein is injected with a very fine needle.

- How does it feel? Slightly painful; sometimes warmth is felt.

- How long does it take? About fifteen minutes.

- How long before it heals? Swelling may last for up to a month. You must avoid hot drinks, alcohol, spicy foods and exercise for several days following treatment.

- When will I see results? The veins may look more prominent for up to two months (gradually fading over that time).

- How long will it last? Results should be permanent but there is always the chance that new veins will develop and become problematic.

- Any side effects? Bruising and swelling are common. Other complications are rare but can include blistering, burning, inflammation, ulcers, scarring, uneven pigmentation.

- Contraindications? Pregnancy and breastfeeding, diabetes, photosensitivity (or taking photosensitising medication or herbs), sunburn or recent tanning, very dark skin.

- Most suitable age to have it? Any age.

- Cost? Low to medium – varies depending on area treated.

We say: A very long-established treatment. It's reliable and gives good predictable results.

HANDS

Don't forget about your hands; they can give away your age as much (if not more) than your face and neck. As we age, the skin on our hands becomes thinner making veins and joints appear more prominent. Fortunately we can now make hands look young and plumper once more. Generally we tend to use Fat Transplant to give a natural 'hand lift'.

Going deeper: more radical resurfacing (without surgery)

It may sound extreme, but by removing the top layer or layers of skin, you can actually persuade the skin to rejuvenate itself. There is now a huge range of procedures on offer: the traditional forms of resurfacing are chemical peels and dermabrasion/microdermabrasion; these have now been joined by laser treatments and new alternatives such as Exoderm or the moulding mask.

On the whole these are much more invasive strategies than those we have discussed up until now. You should expect to take time off work for recovery and expect some pain and discomfort with many of the procedures. However, the results can be outstanding, literally uncovering an entire new face in many cases.

Which is best? It's a tough question and every surgeon will have their preferred treatment. Old techniques such as dermabrasion and deep phenol peels had good results but the downtime was considerable. Nowadays people can't afford to spend a week off work with a mask over their face waiting for new skin to grow. So the industry has been looking for alternatives that give equally good results but don't require such extensive downtime. That's why treatments such as IPL and Thermage (which we have already discussed) are exciting, as they offer good results without being invasive. We're also very excited about the new Fraxel laser that is far less traumatic to the skin than the old-school lasers.

Out of all the resurfacing treatments, however, we tend to recommend chemical peels. They are, on the whole, less aggressive and also far less dependent on the operator for good results. Laser resurfacing and dermabrasion require considerable skill on the part of the operator. If you go too deep you can easily create scars, micropigmentation and hyperpigmentation. Peels, on the other hand, work by the chemical action of the acid; you know precisely how deep they will penetrate the skin and there is far less margin for error.

Having said that, lasers and IPL can be very effective if you need to treat a specific area or problem. Peels, by their very nature, treat the entire face.

CHEMICAL PEELS

Peels have had some bad press in the past. They left your skin bright red and raw, as if you'd fallen asleep on a sunbed for a few hours. They were akin to dousing your face in an acid bath, and you'd have to go through several weeks of flaking, sore, rough skin before you sloughed off the old skin. Even after you lost that initial burned-to-a-crisp look, the skin could remain extremely red for many months afterwards.

But times and procedures change and now we use a variety of peels in our practice with outstanding results. The basic idea is that you replace the outer (effectively dead) layers of tired, sallow, blemished and wrinkly skin to reveal the fresher, younger-looking layers that lie beneath. This is done by simply painting on a chemical which causes the surface skin layer or layers to be shed. A new healthy, less blotchy skin layer is formed. Quite apart from this re-growth, the added advantage is that the dermis is also jolted into producing new collagen.

There are a host of different peels, from light through to deep peels. A good cosmetic surgeon should be able to guide you to find the one that's right for your skin. We've already seen the minimal superficial peel as a lunchtime procedure. Now let's see what else is on offer.

What is used in a peel?

Pretty much the same chemicals are used in all peels. What varies is the strength of the solution. These are the ones you are most likely to come across:

- **Alpha-hydroxy acid**: a blanket term for a range of acids, derived from natural sources. Usually used for more superficial peels. You will also come across many of these as ingredients in DIY treatments and beauty salon treatments.

  - **citric acid**: derived from citrus fruit. Used in very superficial peels.
  - **malic acid**: derived from apples. Used in very superficial peels.
  - **tartaric acid**: derived from grape extract. Used in very superficial peels.
  - **glycolic acid**: derived from sugar cane. The most commonly used alpha-hydroxy acid in superficial peels. Frequently used to exfoliate the epidermis and stimulate collagen growth. Repeated glycolic acid peels actually strengthen and thicken the skin, and can cut down on uneven pigmentation.
  - **lactic acid**: derived from either sour milk or bilberries. Often used for sensitive skins where glycolic acid is too strong.

- **Trichloroacetic acid (TCA)**: used mainly in medium-depth peels in various strengths. It removes the outer layers of the skin and penetrates the dermis, promoting collagen and elastin regeneration. A good choice for removing fine lines, moderate skin damage, uneven pigmentation. You will require an anaesthetic cream before treatment and cool fans will relieve the burning sensation.

- **Beta-hydroxy acid (salicylic acid)**: used in varying concentrations. This is used in medium-depth peels. It is often used for acne damage and wart removal as well as sun-damaged skin. It is not suitable for very sensitive skin.

- **Resorcinol**: a derivative of phenol that encourages flaking and also helps drive other ingredients further into the skin. Often combined with other acids to deepen results.

- **Phenol**: the original chemical used for deep surgical peels. It uses carbolic acid for deep facial exfoliation. It requires sedation as it penetrates deep into the dermis, causing quite severe trauma. However it is a highly effective treatment for crow's feet, forehead lines, lines around the mouth, upper lip lines, uneven pigmentation and severe sun damage.

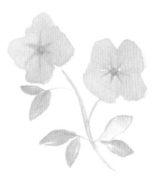

COMBINATION PEELS

Many peels use a combination of chemicals and techniques; these are some you may come across.

- Jessner's Peel: a superficial to medium-depth peel made from a combination of salicylic acid, lactic acid and resorcinol. It is used in varying strengths depending on the amount of damage your skin has. Expect to peel and flake for about a week and then turn pink or brown before your new skin is revealed.

- Obagi Blue Peel: a type of TCA peel that can be used on all skin types, and works well for fine lines and wrinkles, uneven pigmentation and sun damage. Expect your skin to turn blueish following treatment, so you will need to take a few days off work. This peel is particularly useful for darker skins.

- Bio-Medic MicroPeel: a combination of deep exfoliation, an alpha-hydroxy peel and finally cryotherapy in which the surface cells are frozen and removed to reveal fresh smooth skin.

- Moulding Mask: a complex procedure in which the formula is applied to the face, which is then covered with small strips of silk moulded to the contours of the face. The mask is left on for thirty-two to thirty-eight hours and, during that time, the patient should not speak in order to keep the facial muscles inert. The procedure is then repeated periodically over the next few days – usually up to seven days but it can be ten (still using the facial muscles as little as possible; food is liquidised for example). It's a very time-consuming procedure but does have good results.

FACTFILE: MEDIUM-DEPTH PEELS

- What are they good for? Sun-damaged skin, superficial wrinkles, precancerous lesions, patchy/uneven skin, melasma, age spots, active acne and superficial acne scarring.

- What happens? Skin is thoroughly cleansed. Then the active peel solution is applied to the face. In many peels the peel is then removed and the skin is left alone to flake and peel for several days. In others it will be left to work for several hours or even days.

- How does it feel? Expect a burning sensation, mild discomfort and itching.

- How long does it take? From five to thirty minutes, depending on the type of peel.

- How long before it heals? Expect flaking, peeling and scabbing for around a week. Swelling usually subsides after a few days or a week.

- When will I see results? A week to ten days.

- How long will it last? About six to twelve months (most surgeons recommend a course of several treatments).

- Any side effects? Initially you will experience swelling, redness and scabbing. There is a slight risk of infection, scarring or hyperpigmentation (treated areas turn overly pale).

- Contraindications? Peels are not suitable for people on acne drugs (e.g. Roaccutane) and steroids. They are not generally suitable for dark skin (with the exception of Obagi peels).

- Most suitable age to have it? Generally thirties and forties.

- Cost? Medium.

We say: Medium-depth peels are a very effective tool for ironing out moderate skin damage. We use the MY Weekend Peel which works in a slightly different way to most medium-depth peels in that it is applied and then left on to work actively on the skin for seventy-two hours (hence the name – most people choose to have it done just before the weekend so they can relax and experience the optimum benefits). It's not a very deep peel and so can't, with all honesty, deal with serious damage but it does work extremely well for people with sun-damaged skin, superficial wrinkles, pre-cancerous lesions, patchy or uneven skin, melasma (dark patches or age spots), active acne and superficial acne scars.

FACTFILE: DEEP PEELS

- What are they good for? Severe acne scarring, deep dermal pits (large pores), pigmentation changes (including freckles and sunspots), premature skin ageing, severe wrinkling, skin laxity. They are also very useful following a facelift if wrinkles and poor skin quality remain.

- What happens? You are given light sedation and painkillers to eliminate the characteristic burning sensation. The peel solution is applied to the skin where it produces a white blanching, or frosting. When this happens the area is rubbed dry. A red-greyish colour appears instead and the skin becomes swollen. The procedure is normally performed twice. Then the face is covered with airtight tape to form a mask. This is usually removed after about twenty-four hours and replaced with a regenerative mask.

- How does it feel? Your skin can feel very hot and quite sore; many people find the process and after-effects pretty painful. The look of your face can also be quite distressing.

- How long does it take? About two hours, but you may need to remain in hospital overnight.

- How long before it heals? Around one to three weeks (strong sunblock must be worn for about six months after treatment).

- When will I see results? You should notice a difference once the initial shedding of the external skin layers has finished but it takes about three to four months following the peel to notice the full benefits.

- How long will it last? Up to ten years.

- Any side effects? You will have a feeling like a strong sunburn or windburn directly after treatment. Skin will be very red and sore. There is a small risk of infection, scarring and hyperpigmentation as with other peels.

- Contraindications? Peels are not suitable for people on acne drugs (e.g. Roaccutane) and steroids. They are not suitable for dark skin.

- Most suitable age to have it? Forties plus (or earlier for acne scarring, severe sun damage).

- Cost? High.

We say: We use a deep peel called Exoderm that was developed in 1986 to provide a complete and unique solution for ageing skin. The peel is composed of twelve components, including phenol, resorcinol, citric acid and a variety of natural oils. More than a decade of experience in over 10,000 patients and fifteen countries has shown that the method is safe. The results are impressive and produce a high degree of satisfaction. We are confident about recommending Exoderm but if you are considering any other deep peel then do ensure you get all the information, research data and talk to other patients who have had the procedure.

GOLDEN RULES FOR PEELS

1 Follow instructions. Before a peel you may be asked to prepare your skin, using preparations such as gentler alpha-hydroxy acids, Retin A or Hydroquinone. Follow any instructions to the letter; they will increase the effectiveness of your peel and lessen the chance of uneven pigmentation.

2 Do NOT pick or pull at peeling or flaking skin: you could cause scarring or an infection.

3 You will be given specific ointments, moisturisers, lotions and sunblock to use following your peel. Do not use your standard moisturisers or serums as they may diminish the effect of your peel.

4 Avoid the sun if you can and use a high sunblock if you do have to go out in it.

5 Don't even think of any kind of exfoliation treatment or products following a peel.

6 Arnica can help the healing process without decreasing the effectiveness of your peel.

7 Be patient. This is a process that takes time before you see results.

CASE STUDY

Lesley Strickley, forty-eight, lives in Birmingham.

I'm a lively person, full of zest – I'm game for anything. But when I looked in the mirror I just couldn't see that person any more. I looked tired and gaunt. I just felt 'this isn't me'. Part of it was my own fault: I'd become addicted to sunbeds and my skin was awful, terribly dry and if I stopped using the sunbeds it went grey. When I got to my mid-forties, I thought, I've got to stop this.

I had seen Roberto and Maurizio on television a few years before and immediately liked them. I did about a year's worth of research and saw a few surgeons but as soon as I met Roberto I knew he was the one. He was so calm and reassuring. I honestly thought I'd need a face lift or surgery on my eyelids, but Roberto said we needed to sort out the condition of my skin and suggested Exoderm. I looked into it and thought it seemed ideal as I wanted something permanent, something deep that would affect the collagen and give me a slight lift as well as improving my skin tone.

I didn't feel nervous as I was so confident about Roberto. I just knew he wouldn't hurt me – and he didn't. It's a strange procedure though. First the solution is painted on and then you have little plasters stuck all over your face. I had to stay in London overnight and go back to the Centre the next day to have the plasters taken off. The old skin is scraped away which sounds horrible – but you don't feel anything. Then you have this powder put on your face and it sets to a green mask. I felt a bit like the Hulk and you do have to chop up your food for a week as the mask is so stiff. It throbbed a little bit after about three days but that soon wore off. On the eighth day you put on Vaseline to soften the mask so you can take it off. My skin was a little pink – as if I'd been in the sun – but I could wear make-up and the pinkness didn't last long.

The results got better and better over the next few months, as the skin made new collagen and elastin. Now it's fabulous – bright and plump and smooth. I've lost all the small wrinkles around my eyes and some deeper ones down my cheeks too. Best of all, it's given me such huge confidence. I used to wear make-up to cover up my looks; now I enjoy wearing it to enhance them. Recently I did a catwalk show for charity and felt fabulous. I'd never have done that before. People say I look younger than my age and often think I'm in my mid-thirties, which also gives your confidence a boost. It's like being given a second chance and I'd recommend it to anyone.

LASER TREATMENT

If you don't like the sound of having acid applied to your skin, laser resurfacing might be more to your liking. There are basically two kinds of resurfacing: ablative and non-ablative. Ablative is the most invasive, and involves passing a laser over the area to be treated, directly removing the outer layer of the skin. This will cause obvious skin damage, with the skin appearing red and weeping, before crusting over, scabbing and flaking (and finally sloughing off to reveal fresh new skin). The most common kind of ablative laser is the CO_2 (carbon dioxide) laser, which really can resurface the skin in the manner of a deep phenol peel or dermabrasion, but it's a tough procedure. Many lasers are very specialised, and will target a specific problem, such as melanin or the dyes used for tattoos.

The very latest laser treatments, however, are non-ablative and much less invasive. They involve firing a beam at your skin, creating damage only in the lower layers of the skin (predominantly the dermis), while leaving the outer layers (the epidermis) untouched. This prompts the skin to produce collagen to repair the problem and, as a side effect, skin texture is improved and rejuvenated. It may sound a bit scary, but modern procedures are very careful in their approach and it's actually much less invasive and traumatic than medium to deep peels and dermabrasion. Because all the work is happening at a deeper level, you will only experience very minor swelling or pinkness, and will usually require very little downtime.

Just to confuse matters there is now a new form of laser treatment, the Fraxel laser, which can be considered to lie right in between the ablative and non-ablative lasers in that it works in vertical lines through the skin. It's an exciting new development.

Laser treatment is generally good for getting rid of (or lessening) acne scarring, sun damage, age spots, uneven pigmentation, fine lines and wrinkles, scars and stretch marks, birthmarks and port-wine stains, warts and tattoos. It also boosts your collagen production making skin generally plumper, brighter and healthier-looking.

Types of laser

ABLATIVE LASERS

- **Carbon dioxide (CO2) laser/Ultrapulse:** light is directed at the skin and is attracted to the water contained in it; the water absorbs the light and removes damage from the skin. Its effects are comparable to those of a deep phenol peel. This can be a painful option with a long period of recovery needed (the skin will remain red or pink for up to three months). It used to be commonly used but is now treated with caution as usually there are far less invasive options available to achieve the same results. It also carries the risk of scarring and hyperpigmentation, particularly in people with darker skin.

- **Erbium laser:** a more moderate form of the CO2 laser, its effects are comparable to a medium-depth peel, such as a TCA peel. It'll still take about a month before the redness subsides.

- **Pigment lasers:** used to remove sunspots, liver spots, freckles and tattoos. Scabs form and will take up to a month to go. Redness will persist for up to several months.

- **Vascular lasers**: specifically target rosacea, dilated or broken blood vessels, spider or thread veins. The laser homes in on the haemoglobin within the vessel and removes redness. This form of treatment rarely requires any downtime.

MID-WAY LASER

- **Fraxel laser**: a selective laser that produces microscopic columns of skin damage. Your skin is prompted to repair itself by producing collagen. See below.

NON-ABLATIVE LASERS

- **Cool Touch/Smooth Beam**: heats the area between the epidermis and the dermis, stimulating collagen production and correcting wrinkles from the inside out. A cryogen (freezing) spray is applied before treatment, cooling the epidermis and letting the laser penetrate to the warmer level required.

- **NLite**: yellow light passes through the epidermis and stimulates new collagen production in the dermis. Effective for wrinkles.

FACTFILE: FRAXEL LASER

- How does it work? It fires a laser beam at your face, producing microscopic columns of skin damage. Your skin is prompted to repair itself by producing collagen.

- What's it good for? Acne scarring, sun damage, age spots, uneven pigmentation, lines and wrinkles on face, neck, chest and hands.

- What happens? You are given a local anaesthetic. A tint is applied to the skin, darkening the surface and showing up tiny folds needing treatment. An optical tracking system targets the tinted folds.

- How does it feel? Warm, maybe a tiny bit uncomfortable.

- How long does it take? About forty to forty-five minutes. You will need about four treatments, at weekly or fortnightly intervals.

- How long before it heals? Forty-eight hours to a week.

- When will I see results? After a week.

- How long will it last? Up to ten years.

- Any side effects? Puffiness, swelling and a feeling of heat (like a mild sunburn). Skin may stay slightly red or swollen for up to a week. Skin will naturally exfoliate, flaking rather like that following sunburn.

- Contraindications? Avoid sunbathing and sunbeds for several weeks before treatment.

- Most suitable age to have it? Twenties for acne scarring, thirties plus for skin rejuvenation.

- Cost? High.

We say: A very exciting development in laser therapy. One of the best lasers we've seen and experienced.

GOLDEN RULES FOR LASER RESURFACING

1   Find a surgeon who really understands lasers and can suggest the very best for your needs. This is a huge and technical field, so choose carefully.

2   Ask if you need a spot test. Most laser procedures require this as it's an effective way to find out how your skin will react.

3   Check out your ethnic background several generations back. This may sound strange but laser resurfacing can produce uneven pigmentation in people with dark skins (and even a grandparent with a darker skin tone could affect your outcome). If in doubt, have a spot test.

4   Tell your surgeon your entire medical and surgical history (including non-invasive and topical skin treatments).

5   Talk the options over with your surgeon. Consider whether you would be better off with another form of resurfacing (peels or dermabrasion).

6   Never pick at scabs, flakes or peeling skin. This can cause infection and possibly scarring.

7   Follow instructions. You will probably be given special creams, ointments and possibly bandages. Don't use anything on your skin that has not been cleared by your surgeon.

8   Protect your skin from the sun. New skin is very susceptible to sun damage so you need to keep out of it for several months. If you do go out, always use sunblock.

DERMABRASION

Dermabrasion was originally developed in the 1950s when it was used to treat facial scarring, whether from accidents or from acne or chickenpox. While it is still used for this purpose, it is also a useful tool for treating moderate to deep facial lines and wrinkles, severe sun damage and uneven pigmentation. Basically the procedure removes the top layer of skin – just as a chemical peel or laser resurfacing does. The difference is that while a chemical peel uses a caustic chemical solution to dissolve the top layer and laser treatment uses, well, a laser, dermabrasion uses surgical instruments to rub away the layer. It's akin to sanding down a door, removing the top level of varnish and grime.

Generally speaking, dermabrasion is used for deeper lines and scarring than chemical peels, but it really depends greatly on your individual skin and problem. Most cosmetic surgeons will be experienced in both kinds of procedure and will be able to advise you on the best choice. One good point about this form of resurfacing: it is particularly useful for people with darker skin, as there is less risk of the discolouration that can happen with other procedures.

FACTFILE: DERMABRASION

- Other names: Dermaplaning.

- How does it work? The top layers of skin are sanded away by an abrasive material (a rapidly spinning wheel, blade or wire brush), stimulating new skin to grow in its place.

- What's it good for? Medium to deep facial lines and wrinkles, severe sun damage, uneven pigmentation, acne (and other) scarring.

- What happens? You take tretinoin cream for two to three weeks before treatment to lessen the time needed for new skin growth. You will be given an anaesthetic (either general or local). First your skin is thoroughly cleaned and a numbing spray may be applied to freeze and firm the surface being treated. Your surgeon will then apply the dermabrasion tool over the area, carefully removing layers of skin until reaching the optimum level (where the scar or wrinkle will be less visible). A compress will be applied to reduce side effects and speed up healing.

- How does it feel? The treatment itself is not painful as you are sedated but you should expect a fair degree of tingling, burning and stinging afterwards. Some people find the after-treatment period very uncomfortable or even painful. Your face will also itch as new skin grows: think back to when you scabbed a knee when you were a child.

- How long does it take? It depends on the area being treated: from a few minutes for scars right up to two hours for a large area of face.

- How long before it heals? New skin usually grows after a week to ten days. It will take up to three months before full healing is complete. You should expect to be off work for about two weeks.

- When will I see results? After a month to six weeks.

- How long will it last? Providing you stick to a healthy lifestyle the effects are quite long-lasting – up to around ten years.

- Any side effects? Initially there will be swelling, redness, itching, burning and stinging. Yellow crusting or scabs can be signs of infection (see your surgeon). Persistent redness could indicate a scar is forming (see your surgeon). Occasional side effects include scarring, infection, blistering, herpes simplex infection, discolouration. You will need to keep out of the sun and apply a broad-spectrum sunscreen daily for six to twelve months following treatment to prevent unwanted pigmentation.

- Contraindications? Pregnancy, breastfeeding. Active herpes infection. Patients with a history of keloid formation will need to have a spot test. If you are having treatment with isotretinoin, you will need to wait up to twelve months before treatment. Skin diseases such as acne, rosacea and dermatitis may flare up following treatment. People with a history of herpes, impetigo, and cold sores will need antibiotic medication to prevent flare-ups. Some surgeons will be unwilling to treat you if you have had radiation treatment and dermabrasion may be contraindicated if you have had a chemical peel previously.

- Most suitable age to have it? Any age for scarring. Otherwise, mid-thirties plus.

- Cost? Medium.

We say: This was a good treatment and it still has a place in cosmetic surgery. In our practice we sometimes use it in association with a deep peel, for instance where there is a large amount of deep acne scarring.

Chapter Eight

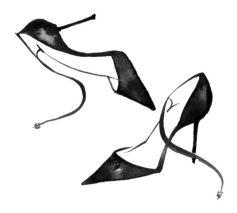

The big change

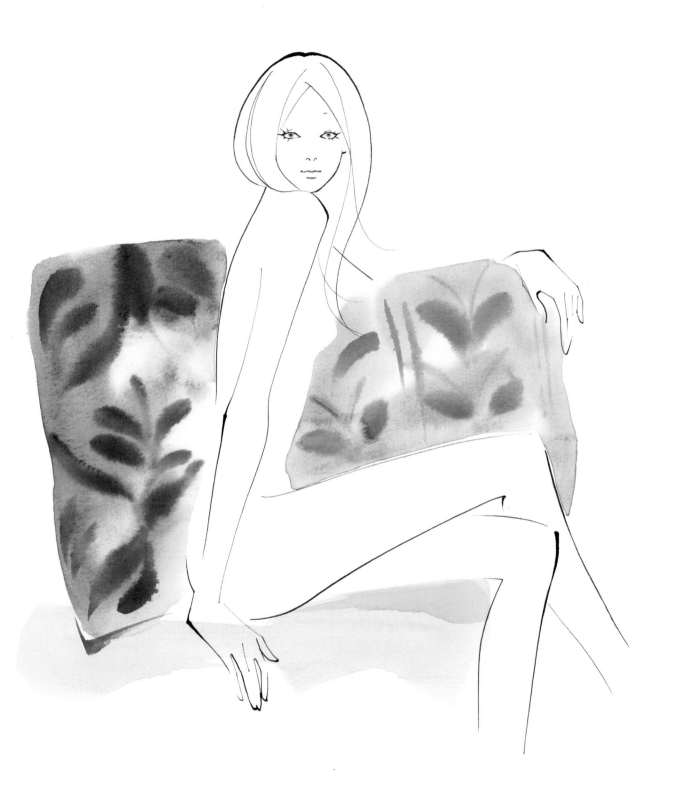

So you have decided you want major cosmetic surgery? It's a big decision but hundreds of thousands of women would say it's the best one they ever made. You can do a huge amount with the Natural Rejuvenation Plan and non-invasive or less invasive procedures can work wonders too, but sometimes you just can't beat the results you get with surgery. It could be that nature has dealt you a tough hand, and there's nothing diet and exercise can do to boost a tiny bust or trim down an ungainly nose. Sometimes, even when you have followed all the diet and exercise advice to the letter, you are still left with stubborn chunks of fat that simply won't fall into line. Having children often leaves women with sagging breasts and aprons of flabby skin, denting confidence and turning them into truly desperate housewives. These are the times when cosmetic surgery really does come into its own.

As we've already said, this isn't about vanity. It's about giving you back the confidence you should have as your birthright. It's about making life feel good, about letting you wear what you want (or letting you strip off without worrying).

In this section we'll outline the major procedures and what to expect from them. We'll tell you what is possible and what isn't. Take your time making your decision and finding the right surgeon to perform your procedure – this isn't something to rush.

The Top Ten Surgical Procedures
According to the British Association of Aesthetic Plastic Surgeons (BAAPS) these are currently the most popular surgical procedures.

1   Breast augmentation

2   Blepharoplasty (eyelid surgery)

3   Breast reduction

4   Face/neck lift

5   Rhinoplasty (nose job)

6   Abdominoplasty (tummy tuck)

7   Liposuction (major)

8   Otoplasty (ear pinning)

9   Liposuction (minor)

10 Brow lift

Our Top Ten Surgical Procedures

In our practice we see a slightly different picture. Our top ten procedures are as follows:

1   Liposuction/LipoSelection

2   Breast augmentation

3   Face/neck lift

4   Fat harvesting/transplant

5   Blepharoplasty

6   Rhinoplasty

7   Breast reduction

8.   Abdominoplasty

9   Otoplasty

10   Brow lift

However, it's worth pointing out that, as often happens, statistics don't really show the true picture. The most common treatment of all is not actually surgical – it is, in fact, botulinum toxin injections.

Risks

A note on complications/side effects: as we have already explained, all surgery carries risks. Although, in the hands of a good surgeon, cosmetic surgery is usually perfectly safe, we have to point out that very occasionally things can go wrong. The major risks from cosmetic surgery are exactly the same as those you would expect from any other type of surgery. Just to be completely clear and ethical, we will repeat the risks once more; but do remember these are rare and extreme.

- Temporary paralysis
- Nerve damage
- Blood clot, possibly leading to stroke or embolism
- Bleeding, haematoma
- Brain damage
- Airway obstruction
- Abnormal heart rhythm
- Heart attack
- Excessive scarring
- Puckering or dimpling of the skin
- Perforation of internal organs
- Post-operative numbness
- Infection

We will not outline these risks in the factfiles for each procedure, but please note they do apply to every surgical procedure.

Contraindications

There are certain people who should not have particular forms of surgery. Where contraindications exist for specific procedures we will list them in the factfile for each procedure. However there are some general contraindications for the majority of procedures. These are:

- Pregnancy
- Severe medical conditions, such as active cancer, blood disorders, severe epilepsy. However each case should be judged individually – consult your surgeon for advice.
- Psychological disorders
- Unrealistic expectations
- Heavy smoking

Cost

Prices will vary enormously across the country and in individual clinics. We have however tried to give an indication of price, as follows:

- *Low: under £1,000*
- *Medium: up to £3,000*
- *High: £3,000 plus*

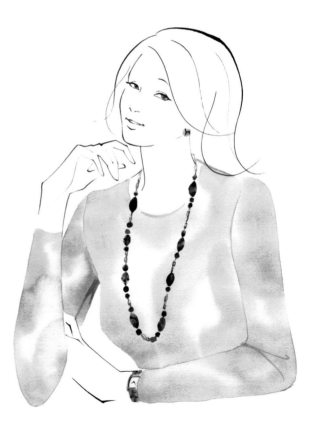

The Face and Neck

FACELIFTS

The face and neck are the parts of the body most exposed to the elements and so most affected by the ageing process. Exposure to the sun, a less than healthy lifestyle and the passing of time itself can lead to sagging and bagging, wrinkles, lines and generally jaded, tired-looking skin. In the past we just had to grin (or weep) and bear it, accepting our fate and ageing as gracefully (and with as good grace) as we could manage. Then along came facelifts and the age of the Hollywood horror was born. Facelifts were synonymous with taut, tight, wind-tunnel faces and rictus smiles. Only the truly desperate followed suit. Now, of course, it's all very different. There are a range of lifts for every face: subtle, natural, safe. It's purely a question of which one would suit you best. Let's look at the options.

WHICH FACELIFT?

TYPE OF FACELIFT	CLASSIC	MACS	THREAD LIFT
Ideal age	55+	40s–50s	30s
Amount of tautness/tone provided	***	**	*
Subtlety/natural look provided	*	**	***
Neck improvement	***	**	*

As you will see, the thread lift will give the most natural, subtle effect but will not be suitable for older patients who have a lot of loose skin.

FACTFILE: CLASSIC FACELIFT/ENDOSCOPIC FACELIFT

- What does it do? Gives a much more youthful appearance by removing excess skin, fat and furrows, tautening up sagging cheeks and tweaking up a downturned smile. It helps to alleviate hoods and bags under the eyes; relieves the deep grooves that may form from nose to mouth, and improves the contours of the neck and jawline.

- Type of anaesthetic? General (very occasionally local).

- Length of stay? Overnight.

- What happens? In the classic facelift a cut is made in the hairline, behind the ear. The skin and muscle are pulled up and back and any excess skin is trimmed away. The surgeon then sutures the wound and applies a dressing. Alternatively an endoscope fitted with a tiny fibre-optic camera may be inserted through small cuts in the mouth and temple; the camera allows the surgeon to see his progress under the skin.

- How does it feel? You should expect pain and discomfort for several days and possibly numbness for several weeks.

- How long does it take? The operation lasts between three and five hours.

- Scars? Yes. Permanent scarring at the side of the face, but it's generally hidden in the hairline and will fade over time.

- Swelling and bruising? Yes. Swelling and bruising can last for several weeks.

- Recovery time? Stitches are removed about a week after surgery. You will be off work for ten to fourteen days. You must avoid strenuous exercise for about two months after surgery.

- Side effects? Complications are rare but the side effects of general surgery are possible. Also, an asymmetrical outcome is possible.

- Contraindications? General.

- When will I see results? After a few months.

- What's the optimum age to have this? Most facelifts are carried out from the ages of forty to sixty, although good results are seen on older faces, providing bone structure is good and skin retains some elasticity.

- Any other procedures to have at the same time? Brow lift, eyelid lift.

- How long will the results last? Between five and ten years, depending on age. The younger you are, the longer the effects will last. It can be repeated if necessary.

- Cost? High.

We say: This is a classic technique that is still an excellent choice for older patients with lots of sagging skin on the face and neck. However it does involve a longer recovery time than other facelifts and gives a less natural look.

FACTFILE: MACS LIFT (MINIMAL ACCESS CRANIAL SUSPENSION)

- Other names: S lift; Short Scar facelift; Mini facelift.

- What does it do? Lifts and refreshes the lower two-thirds of the face (from the temples to lower neck) by lifting the skin and tightening the muscle bands and the layers of tissue connected to the facial muscles. Only a limited amount of skin needs to be removed, leaving nothing but an inconspicuous scar either inside the ear or in the crease in front of the ear and in the hairline above the ear.

- Type of anaesthetic? In contrast to most other techniques, this type of facelift can be performed with local anaesthetic under light sedation. However you may prefer a general anaesthetic.

- Length of stay? Two hours after surgery (for local anaesthetic); overnight (for general).

- What happens? The surgeon makes an S-shaped incision around (or inside) the ear and into the hairline. Soft tissue and muscle is tightened, excess fat and skin are removed and the wound is closed.

- How does it feel? Expect your face to feel swollen, bruised and stiff for quite a few days.

- How long does it take? Surgery takes around two to three hours.

- Scars? Yes, but scarring is minimal and hidden behind or inside the ear and in the hairline.

- Swelling and bruising? Yes, but less than with a classic facelift.

- Recovery time? Around ten days so you will need to take at least a week off work, but all the swelling won't disappear until one month later.

- Side effects? Complications are rare but can include the usual dangers associated with any surgery. You might get an asymmetrical result. Scarring can be visible if not performed well.

- Contraindications? General.

- When will I see results? About two weeks after surgery.

- What's the optimum age to have this? Usually from mid-thirties to fifties.

- Any other procedures to have at the same time? Eye lift, brow lift, chin restructuring.

- How long will the results last? Around five to ten years. It can be repeated if necessary.

- Cost? High.

We say: We like this lift a lot. It's far less invasive than a classic facelift and offers great results with a far swifter recovery time. It gives a very natural result.

However it's not suitable for older patients.

FACTFILE: THREAD LIFT

- Other names: Feather lift, Aptos lift, Contour lift.

- What does it do? Remodels and rejuvenates sagging skin without the need for scars and invasive surgery. It lifts up saggy brows, opens up the eyes (often eliminating the need for blepharoplasty, eyelid surgery). It also lifts and tightens a sagging jawline.

- Type of anaesthetic? Local or IV sedation.

- Length of stay? One to two hours after surgery.

- What happens? Threads are inserted with a fine needle; a typical face will need around twelve to sixteen threads around the brow, mid-face and neck. Your own collagen will surround the threads and maintain the effect. There are two major types of thread – see below.

- How does it feel? Expect some discomfort but no real pain.

- How long does it take? About one hour.

- Scars? Minimal. There may be some tiny scars at the injection sites but these will fade with time.

- Swelling and bruising? Yes, some but ice compresses are recommended for the first couple of days to minimise this.

- Recovery time? You will need to take a week off work.

- Side effects? Complications are rare but include the usual dangers of any surgery. Sometimes free-floating threads pucker or protrude, or come loose – but this can easily be remedied. Asymmetry is possible. Puckering and skin folds are possible.

- Contraindications? General.

- When will I see results? After about seventy-two hours.

- What's the optimum age to have this? From about thirty to fifty.

- Any other procedures to have at the same time? Fat injection, lip enhancement.

- How long will the results last? Two to three years. You can repeat or reverse the procedure at any time.

- Cost? Medium.

We say: Worth while for younger patients who do not want or need an extreme lift. It's a good technique and the results are natural and impressive. The downside is that it isn't long-lasting. It is also a valid alternative for heavy smokers as this is one of the few procedures for which heavy smoking is not contraindicated. It's also useful for buying time while waiting for more aggressive procedures later in life.

Which Threads?

There are two major kinds of threads used in a Thread lift. We tend to use contour or suspension threads.

1. Free-floating threads: Aptos threads are the best known of this type. They work by traction, pulling the skin into place. The threads have barbs. Once the thread is in place, the surgeon pulls it and the barbs tug the skin into place. Any ends are cut off. The threads remain permanently under the skin.

   Advantages: an easier, more straightforward procedure requiring less skill from the surgeon.

   Disadvantages: may slip, protrude or be visible under the skin. Results are shorter-lasting and may not be as dramatic.

2. Suspension or contour threads: these also come in various types: prolene or nylon, absorbable or non-absorbable. They are hooked or sutured on to a stable structure on the face or scalp and then the skin is gently pulled up into its new position.

   Advantages: results are longer-lasting, more dramatic and there is less risk of threads coming loose, protruding or being visible.

   Disadvantages: more demanding technique requiring far more skill on the part of the surgeon. Relapse is possible.

FACTFILE: BROW LIFT

- Other names: Forehead lift.

- What does it do? Subtly lifts the forehead and eyebrows to remove lines, wrinkles and sagging skin.

- Type of anaesthetic? General or sedation.

- Length of stay? One night.

- What happens? A classic brow lift involves one long incision being made from ear to ear (usually just behind the natural hairline), after which the surgeon pulls up the muscles and excess skin. An alternative is the endoscopic brow lift in which several inch-long incisions are made (again in the hairline) and the surgeon uses an endoscope with a telescopic camera attached so they can watch progress under the skin. The skin is pulled up, muscles removed or loosened, and eyebrows lifted and held in place with stitches.

- How does it feel? You should expect pain for a few days and swelling, bruising and numbness for several weeks.

- How long does it take? Two hours.

- Scars? Yes, but scars are usually hidden by hair or the natural creases of the skin; endoscopic scars are even more minimal.

- Swelling and bruising? Yes, swelling and bruising will last for around two weeks.

- Recovery time? You will be off work for about two weeks.

- Side effects? If the stitches are too tight you may get headaches. Numbness lasting for a few weeks is possible (in very rare cases this is permanent). Tightening, swelling and nerve damage usually resolve in a few months. The usual complications connected with any surgery are possible.

- Contraindications? General.

- When will I see results? About two months following surgery.

- What's the optimum age to have this? Fifty to sixty.

- Any other procedures to have at the same time? Many people combine it with a lower facelift. It is possible to reduce the bossing or frontal bone on the forehead to remove a heavy look.

- How long will the results last? Usually around five to ten years.

- Cost? High.

We say: It provides good results but we can now perform a chemical brow lift with botulinum injections or offer a far less invasive option with a thread lift.

FACTFILE: NECK LIFT

- Other names: Platysmaplasty.

- What does it do? Removes sagging skin around the neck and jawline, tightening muscles and skin to create a tauter, more youthful look.

- Type of anaesthetic? General anaesthetic or local with sedation.

- Length of stay? One night or day care if sedation.

- What happens? Incisions are made under the chin and behind or under your ears. Then the surgeon pulls up the muscles and skin, taking away any excess. Liposuction or LipoSelection can be carried out at the same time to remove any fat in the chin.

- How does it feel? You should expect pain for a few days. Swelling, burning, tingling and occasional pain may last for up to three weeks.

- How long does it take? Three hours.

- Scars? Yes, although most scars will be hidden behind the ear and in the folds of your skin.

- Swelling and bruising? Yes, it may take several weeks for swelling to subside entirely.

- Recovery time? Stitches are removed a week after surgery. You will need to rest and be off work for about two weeks.

- Side effects? Puckering, lumpiness and uneven skin tone are possible (but rare). The usual complications for surgery are possible. Asymmetry is possible.

- Contraindications? General.

- When will I see results? Two months following surgery.

- What's the optimum age to have this? Forty plus.

- Any other procedures to have at the same time? Liposuction to remove a double chin. Commonly combined with a facelift.

- How long will the results last? Five to ten years, depending on your skin and age.

- Cost? High.

We say: If you have a very heavy neck this really is the only valid treatment. However for milder cases, a good MACS lift with LipoSelection to the neck will give an equally good result.

FACTFILE: CHEEK AUGMENTATION

- Other names: Cheek implants.

- What does it do? Creates a more youthful appearance by plumping sunken cheeks.

- Type of anaesthetic? Local or sedation.

- Length of stay? Day care.

- What happens? An incision is made inside the mouth or just beneath the lower eyelashes and a permanent implant is positioned over the cheekbone or in the mid-cheek area. See pages 135–142 for information on the various implants.

- How does it feel? It is pretty painful and you should expect to find it hard to talk or smile for several days following surgery.

- How long does it take? Half an hour to two hours.

- Scars? None visible if the incision is inside the mouth; minimal if beneath the lashes.

- Swelling and bruising? Yes, quite considerable but it will ease within a week. Sometimes swelling can continue for a few months. It is common to think you have too much filler – this is often down to post-operative swelling.

- Recovery time? You can return to work two days to a week following surgery.

- Side effects? The usual risks of any surgery. Possible asymmetry.

- Contraindications? General.

- When will I see results? About one month after surgery for best results.

- What's the optimum age to have this? Thirty plus.

- Any other procedures to have at the same time? Facelift.

- How long will the results last? Cheek implants are permanent.

- Cost? Medium.

We say: We much prefer to perform cheek augmentation by fat injection because it is simpler, safer and looks more natural. If you do not have enough fat to harvest, we can use fillers, generally either SubQ (a hyaluronic acid filler) or hydroxyapatite.

FACTFILE: CHEEK REDUCTION

- Other names: Buccal fat removal.

- What does it do? Gives a tighter look to the cheeks and middle face.

- Type of anaesthetic? Local with sedation.

- Length of stay? Day care.

- What happens? An incision is made between the gums and cheek, usually towards the back of the mouth. The surgeon will cut through muscle and remove fat. The incision is closed and sealed with antiseptic gauze.

- How does it feel? Discomfort rather than pain.

- How long does it take? One hour.

- Scars? None visible as they are inside the mouth.

- Swelling and bruising? Yes, there will be swelling and bruising for several weeks after surgery.

- Recovery time? A few days. You should expect discomfort, tingling, burning and sensations of cold for a few weeks and you will need to be very careful when eating and brushing your teeth.

- Side effects? Rarely there may be numbness and puckering of the skin. There may also be the complications that can occur with any surgery.

- Contraindications? General.

- When will I see results? After two weeks.

- What's the optimum age to have this? Any age.

- Any other procedures to have at the same time? Facelift.

- How long will the results last? Five to ten years.

- Cost? Medium.

We say: Personally we do not like to remove fat from the face as we feel it is very ageing. If you want to look younger, our advice is to keep some fat in your face.

FACTFILE: CHIN IMPLANT

- Other names: Mentoplasty.

- What does it do? Helps define lower face by correcting a receding chin.

- Type of anaesthetic? General or sedation.

- Length of stay? Overnight if general, day care if sedation.

- What happens? An incision is made either inside the mouth, on either side of the lower lip, or under the chin. The surgeon will create a pocket into which they will insert the implant. This is stitched into place (usually with dissolvable sutures) and the incision is closed up. There are a variety of implants available, some permanent, some temporary or semi-permanent (see pages 104–12 for details).

- How does it feel? It will be painful for a few days and tender and sore for up to several weeks.

- How long does it take? Ninety minutes.

- Scars? You may have a tiny scar if the incision is made under the chin, but this will fade.

- Swelling and bruising? Yes, swelling and bruising will make talking and smiling painful for several days to a week; they may take several weeks to subside entirely.

- Recovery time? You will be off work for two days to a week.

- Side effects? Temporary numbness of the lower lip is common. Sometimes implants do not fix to the bone and so may feel unstable (this does not usually affect the appearance of the chin). The outline of the implant can sometimes be seen. The chin may crease unnaturally when you smile or grimace. The lower lip may remain permanently numb. Muscles around the mouth may become weakened. Otherwise the usual possible complications of any surgery apply.

- Contraindications? General.

- When will I see results? Usually best results are seen after a couple of months.

- What's the optimum age to have this? Any age.

- Any other procedures to have at the same time? Rhinoplasty.

- How long will the results last? It depends on the implant used: from a year to permanently.

- Cost? Medium.

We say: We prefer to perform genioplasty (chin surgery) in most cases so we can use your own bone. The chin is broken and then repositioned (we can move it up, down, back or forwards) or reshaped. It is not as painful as it sounds! Alternatively we can boost the chin using your own fat or different types of filler.

THE EYES

Bright sparkling eyes are essential for a youthful beautiful look. They are one of the first things other people notice about us. Unfortunately they are one of the most sensitive and hence most easily aged parts of the body. As we get older, the delicate skin around the eyes easily stretches. The upper lids tend to sag giving a drooping or hooded look. Equally, it's common to develop bags under the eyes. Lines and wrinkles add up to a tired and weary appearance. Eye surgery (known as blepharoplasty) is one of the most frequently performed cosmetic enhancements. It involves the removal of bags under the eyes and any excess skin around the eyes, creating a fresh-faced, wide-awake look. Lines and wrinkles are often softened in the process but this is not specifically a wrinkle cure. However, if you are not satisfied with the effect, wrinkles can be further treated with botulinum toxin, IPL, lasers and peels. Eye surgery cannot remove dark circles under the eyes, but dedicated creams or chemical peels can relieve this problem. Finally, do not expect your eye operation to lift sagging eyebrows – for that you will need to combine treatment with a brow lift. For this reason, eye surgery is often performed in conjunction with other facial surgery procedures such as a facelift or brow lift. Nowadays most eye surgery is performed under local anaesthetic or sedation, so you won't need to be admitted to hospital. Sometimes the operation can be performed from the inside of the eyelid, so there is not even temporary scarring.

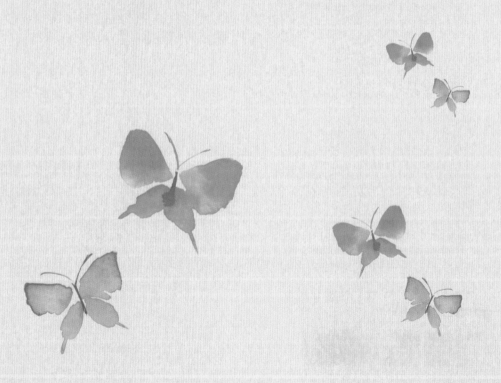

FACTFILE: UPPER BLEPHAROPLASTY

- Other names: Upper eye lift.

- What does it do? Lifts drooping upper eyelids to make eyes look fresh, alert and bright.

- Type of anaesthetic? Local or IV sedation.

- Length of stay? Day care.

- What happens? An incision is made into the natural crease in the eyelid. Excess fat is removed and excess skin and muscle is trimmed away. The incisions are closed up, antiseptic ointment is applied and an ice pack put over the eyes.

- How does it feel? Sore and uncomfortable, rather like being given a black eye. Your eyes may feel gritty, dry and tearful.

- How long does it take? About an hour.

- Scars? There may be a tiny scar in the crease of the eyelid.

- Swelling and bruising? Yes, usually lasting for about ten days.

- Recovery time? Stitches are removed after about three days. You will need to take a week off work. Strenuous exercise must be avoided for three weeks. If you usually wear contact lenses you may need to wear glasses for a few weeks following surgery.

- Side effects? Temporary side effects can include blurred vision, dry sore eyes, increased tear production, problems closing the eyelid. Other rare complications are those common to all surgery. Asymmetry is possible.

- Contraindications? General.

- When will I see results? After about three weeks.

- What's the optimum age to have this? Thirty plus.

- Any other procedures to have at the same time? Many people have a combined upper and lower eye lift. Some people combine it with facelifts.

- How long will the results last? Ten to fifteen years.

- Cost? Medium.

We say: It's very common and very popular with good reason – it's a great procedure. Even when performed on its own it will give you a rejuvenated look.

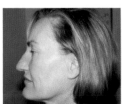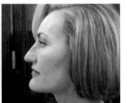

Before   *After*

FACTFILE: LOWER BLEPHAROPLASTY

- Other names: Lower eye recontouring, eyebag removal, lower lid surgery, SOOF lift.

- What does it do? Reduces puffiness and any excess skin under the eyes, giving a fresher younger look.

- Type of anaesthetic? Local anaesthetic or IV sedation.

- Length of stay? Day care.

- What happens? An incision is made under the lower lashes or on the inside of the lower eyelid. Excess fat, skin and muscle is trimmed away and the cut is closed up. The SOOF (sub-orbicularis oculi fat) lift takes the excess fat and positions it behind the muscle, instead of removing it. This stops the eyes looking sunken. After surgery antiseptic ointment is applied followed by an ice pack.

- How does it feel? You will feel a fair amount of soreness and discomfort, rather like having a black eye. Your eyes may feel gritty, dry and sore.

- How long does it take? About an hour.

- Scars? None visible if the incision is made inside the eyelid; otherwise minimal.

- Swelling and bruising? Yes, your eyes will be sore and bruised for several weeks.

- Recovery time? Stitches are removed after three days. You should be off work for about a week. You should not undergo strenuous activity for three weeks. If you usually wear contact lenses you may need to wear glasses for a few weeks following surgery.

- Side effects? Temporary side effects can include excess tear production, sore gritty eyes, blurred vision and dry eyes. Rare complications are those common to all surgery. If too much skin is removed, you may end up with ectropian (the lid being turned away from the eye) and scleral show (when too much of the white is shown under the pupil, giving a very unnatural look).

- Contraindications? General. Also glaucoma, thyroid disease, unilateral blindness, myasthenia gravis.

- When will I see results? After about three months for best results.

- What's the optimum age to have this? Generally thirties plus. However some people have it in their twenties.

- Any other procedures to have at the same time? Commonly performed with upper eyelid surgery; also face and brow lifts.

- How long will the results last? About ten to fifteen years.

- Cost? Medium.

We say: A good technique, very important in facial rejuvenation. It is better to be conservative with this technique to avoid the sunken eye look. Sometimes fat injections to the tear trough could be a simpler and more rewarding alternative.

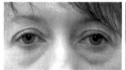 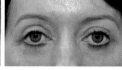

Before   *After*

EARS

Ears can affect the entire balance of a face. Sticking-out ears are often 'pinned' in childhood and we suspect their owners are always mightily relieved their parents took such a step. However many jug ears remain, haunting their owners, into adulthood. No need – otoplasty is a very straightforward procedure that tucks ears back into their rightful place and proportions. Earlobe surgery is also a possibility, repairing and refining overly long or unsightly earlobes. It can also remove lumpy scars that can form after ear piercing. Small things maybe, but they make a large difference.

FACTFILE: OTOPLASTY

- Other names: Ear pinning.

- What does it do? Corrects ears that protrude. While it is most commonly performed on children, this procedure can be very effective on adults as well.

- Type of anaesthetic? Local, usually combined with sedation.

- Length of stay? A couple of hours following surgery.

- What happens? Usually a small incision is made in the back of the ear to expose the ear cartilage. The cartilage is then sculpted and bent back towards the head. Non-removable stitches may be used to help maintain the new shape. Occasionally, a larger piece of cartilage will be removed to provide a more natural-looking fold when the surgery is complete. Another technique involves a similar incision in the back of the ear. Skin is removed and stitches are used to fold the cartilage back on itself to reshape the ear without removing cartilage.

- How does it feel? It may feel a little sore following surgery. As the wound heals your ears might feel as if they are being pulled back, or feel tight.

- How long does it take? One hour.

- Scars? Very small and discreet.

- Swelling and bruising? A small amount is possible.

- Recovery time? You need to have your stitches removed after a week, if they are not absorbable. You should be back to work after a week; for the first week you have to wear an ear band twenty-four hours a day.

- Side effects? The usual risks of any surgery. A very few people develop a blood clot on the ear (which can be removed). Occasionally an infection in the cartilage can cause scar tissue to form.

- Contraindications? General.

- When will I see results? One week after surgery.

- What's the optimum age to have this? Children generally have this performed between the ages of four (when ears are fully formed) and fourteen. Adults any age can have the procedure.

- Any other procedures to have at the same time? On adults, any facial procedures.

- How long will the results last? Permanently.

- Cost? Medium.

We say: A good reliable technique which has great psychological benefits for many patients.

FACTFILE: EARLOBE SURGERY

- What does it do? Repairs torn or cleft earlobes, removes old scarring or reduces the size or protruding nature of the earlobe.

- Type of anaesthetic? Local.

- Length of stay? A few hours.

- What happens? Incisions are made, scarring or tissue may be removed and the formation of the earlobe rearranged to make a pleasing shape.

- How does it feel? You feel nothing during the procedure. Afterwards you may feel a small amount of discomfort.

- How long does it take? Thirty minutes to an hour.

- Scars? Scarring is minimal and usually hidden behind the earlobe.

- Swelling and bruising? Minimal.

- Recovery time? There is no downtime for this procedure, although you will need to avoid getting the earlobe wet for a week and should not wear earrings for at least one month.

- Side effects? Usual risks of any surgery.

- Contraindications? General.

- When will I see results? Once any swelling has subsided (usually seven days).

- What's the optimum age to have this? Any age.

- Any other procedures to have at the same time? Facelift.

- How long will the results last? The results should be permanent. If you are prone to keloids, it is possible future scarring may occur.

- Cost? Medium.

We say: A simple technique that can give back confidence. It also allows the patient to be able to wear earrings again.

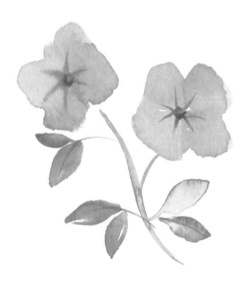

THE NOSE

If you don't like your nose, you're not alone. Absolutely hordes of people are unhappy with the shape of their nose, thinking it too long, too wide or simply plain ugly. If it's any comfort, very few people are born with naturally perfect noses. Time and time again we see patients whose noses are literally ruining their lives, making them feel self-conscious and really denting their confidence. Because the nose sits right in the centre of the face, it's always on display and simply cannot be disguised. No wonder so many people choose surgery.

A new nose won't just make you look good, it could also make you feel much better too. Some noses restrict the airway, giving rise to breathing difficulties or even headaches. So there can be huge health benefits to having rhinoplasty, cosmetic nasal surgery. Rhinoplasty can reduce or increase the size of your nose, change the shape of the tip or the bridge, narrow the span of the nostrils or change the angle between your nose and upper lip. It can also correct birth defects or injuries. A good nose job can transform your face and your self-confidence. It can also make you look years younger. As we grow older and our facial tissue shrinks back, a large nose can suddenly seem much more prominent. A 'beaky' nose is something we sadly often associate with old age. Many people consequently choose to have rhinoplasty alongside or around the same time as a facelift.

Subtlety is key when it comes to noses. This is a very demanding form of surgery and requires true skill and a refined sense of the aesthetic to get exactly the right look. It's absolutely essential you choose a surgeon who has extensive experience and a really good eye for a good nose. Even a fraction of a millimetre can make a huge difference when you're working on a nose. We've all seen what happens when nose jobs go wrong and it's not a pretty sight. Nobody wants a Michael Jackson nose, do they? In the early days of rhinoplasty, it was a case of the smaller the better and you can often tell a 1960s nose by its narrow nostrils and generally tiny size. It's a case of proportion again. A small nose is cute on a child but looks silly on an adult. Most people nowadays are sensible enough to want a nose that is subtly sculpted so it looks totally natural and in perfect proportion to the rest of their features.

Don't forget, either, that it's very common for people to have more than one rhinoplasty. Many people go back for touch-ups and it's much better to under-correct than over-correct. Others will have corrective surgery if their first nose job didn't go far enough or, indeed, went too far. Clever revisional surgery can add back height and width if necessary and can soften irregularities.

FACTFILE: RHINOPLASTY

- Other names: Nose job.

- What does it do? Any number of alterations can be achieved to alter your nose: increasing or decreasing its size, straightening lumps, narrowing nostrils, shifting the overall shape, changing the shape of the tip, altering the angle between the nose and upper lip.

- Type of anaesthetic? General or sedation.

- Length of stay? Day care or overnight (depending on anaesthetic).

- What happens? Surgeons have varying approaches, some preferring a closed procedure (in which the skin is cut inside the rim of the nostrils) while others prefer open procedure (in which an incision is made across the base of the nose). The soft tissue is then separated from the bone and cartilage. The bone may be broken and the cartilage fashioned to create the ideal shape. Fat and tissue can be removed or implants inserted to tailor the shape. After surgery, a splint is put on and the nostrils are packed with antiseptic gauze. Internal incisions are closed with dissolvable stitches while those on the outside will be removed after about a week.

- How does it feel? A dull ache rather than real pain. Breathing can be uncomfortable and you may need to breathe through your mouth for four or five days.

- How long does it take? One or two hours.

- Scars? Most rhinoplasty involves incisions inside the nose so no scarring is visible. There may be minimal scarring if the open tip approach is used (but this fades after around two months and can be covered using make-up in the interim).

- Swelling and bruising? Yes, bruising will last for around two weeks but swelling can persist for several months, especially on the tip of the nose.

- Recovery time? One week, so do plan to take some time off work.

- Side effects? Black eyes are possible if the bone is broken during the procedure. Headaches and nasal bleeding are possible. Lop-sidedness and poor shaping are possible (but repeat surgery is possible). The usual potential risks associated with surgery apply.

- Contraindications? General.

- When will I see results? Usually after three months but the full result can take up to one year to develop. This procedure requires patience.

- What's the optimum age to have this? Any age after the nose has fully developed (around age eighteen).

- Any other procedures to have at the same time? Implants for a weak chin or flat cheekbones. Facelift.

- How long will the results last? Usually results are permanent. Some people opt for further surgery to refine the shape, but you have to wait six months to a year following the first operation.

- Cost? Medium.

We say: Rhinoplasty is one of the oldest and most commonly performed procedures in cosmetic surgery. It is a very rewarding procedure that often has huge psychological benefit to the patient. However it is utterly vital to have a clear understanding of what you want and agree this with your surgeon before surgery.

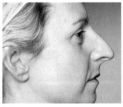

Before

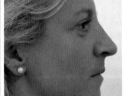

After

CASE STUDY

Arianna de la Cruz, twenty-five, is a teacher from Edinburgh.

I've always hated my nose, even when I was a small child. My brother used to tease me about it endlessly. He inherited my mother's small neat nose while I drew the short straw and ended up with my father's huge one. I always felt that was really unfair as it's OK for men to have 'strong' noses, but on women they're seen as an eyesore.

I had dreamed of rhinoplasty for years but could never afford it. Then two years ago I inherited some money and decided I would fulfil my dream. I knew it wouldn't change my life but I felt it would definitely make me feel more confident and less self-conscious.

Roberto looked carefully at the proportions of my face and said I needed the same nose, but just smaller. That was fine with me – I trusted his judgement. I didn't want it to be horribly obvious I'd had surgery anyhow, I just didn't want my nose to be the first thing people noticed about me!

I was worried about the operation, particularly the fact that I'd have to breathe through my mouth for several days afterwards. I actually practised beforehand and got a bit panicky about it. Also I'm pretty needle-phobic so that bothered me. But truly it was all fine. It went very smoothly and funnily enough the breathing wasn't an issue at all.

It isn't an overnight result. I really would want people to know that. You will find times when you think it's all been a huge mistake and your nose simply isn't the one you wanted. I think everyone goes through that. It does take an awfully long time to settle down and I think mine only really showed its true new shape after about a year. I actually found that first year exciting though – my nose kept getting better and better – but some people could find it frustrating. I would say it's had a huge effect on my personality: I'm much more outgoing and confident now. I can look in the mirror and just see me, not a huge nose attached to a body!

THE LIPS

Everyone wants the perfect pout and now it's relatively simple to get gorgeous luscious lips. Narrowing or thinning of the lips is one of the most obvious signs of ageing, yet it is also one of the simplest problems to solve. We usually recommend injecting filler material such as hyaluronic acid to give a fuller, more youthful look. See pages 135–142 for full details of the range of fillers available. Filler can be injected into one or both lips and also along the upper edge to define the cupid's bow. Once a natural full shape has been achieved, permanent make-up can be used to give added definition. Botulinum can also remove fine lines and lift the corner of the lips.

As we have already explained, we do not ever recommend permanent fillers: we have seen far too many bad reactions ever to sanction their use.

FACTFILE: LIP AUGMENTATION

- Other names: Lip implants.

- What does it do? Plumps and reshapes thin or sagging lips to give a fresh, young, plump-lipped look.

- Type of anaesthetic? Local with a dental block.

- Length of stay? You can leave immediately after surgery.

- What happens? The surgeon will make four tiny incisions into each corner of your mouth and inject or thread the implants into place.

- How does it feel? You should expect some pain following the surgery and possibly numbness and stiffness which makes eating and drinking uncomfortable (this can last for a few days).

- How long does it take? About half an hour.

- Scars? Minimal scarring that is easily concealed with make-up and fades over time.

- Swelling and bruising? Yes, both, sometimes quite severe; swelling can sometimes last for a few days.

- Recovery time? You can normally return to work the same day. Or, if bruising and swelling are severe, you will have to take two or three days off. It takes several weeks for full healing.

- Side effects? Lips can feel stiff, sore and painful. Numbness is also possible. Sometimes the implant will harden or shift, and will need replacing. The usual potential complications for surgery apply.

- Contraindications? Herpes zoster, herpes simplex (cold sores).

- When will I see results? Best results after about a couple of days.

- What's the optimum age to have this? Any age.

- Any other procedures to have at the same time? Botulinum injections.

- How long will the results last? It depends very much on the implant – some are temporary and will last up to a year; others may last longer.

- Cost? Low.

We say: It's a great, easy treatment to have, but don't overdo it. We would also strongly advise you not to have permanent implants or fillers in the lips.

The Body

THE BREASTS

When it comes to breasts, nature never seems to be fair. Only a lucky few women seem to be totally content with the size and shape of their breasts. The majority would rather nature had been more freehanded with her gifts or a little more even-handed: breast asymmetry is a common complaint and a large number of women's breasts vary up to a few cup sizes. Equally, there are plenty of women who wish nature hadn't been quite so generous – overly large breasts can cause as much anguish as tiny ones. Large breasts can invite unwelcome comments and actual physical pain and discomfort: breasts are heavy and running with big breasts can be excruciating. Also, today's fashions are not big breast-friendly and it can be hard to find clothes that hang well on a large-busted frame.

As with most things in life, and particularly in cosmetic surgery, a sense of proportion is required. Beautifully sized and shaped breasts make a woman look and feel womanly, sensual and confident. No wonder breast surgery is so incredibly popular. Look at the back of any women's glossy magazine and you will find page after page of 'perfect' breasts. Beware. While breast augmentation (the traditional 'boob job') is pretty straightforward surgery, there is plenty that can go wrong and we can't count the number of revisions we have had to do for women desperately unhappy with their new breasts.

We can increase the bustline by up to two cup sizes (no more), by inserting an implant behind the breast. Implants can be placed on top of the muscle or behind it – your surgeon will discuss the best method for you.

You can either have the traditional round-shaped implants with high, or super-high profile, or anatomical (breast-shaped) designs. The latest trend is to have slightly asymmetrical breast implants which give a much more natural look. See page 185 for details of the various implants you can have. We would always recommend you try for the most natural look possible. Err on the side of caution and subtlety – you can always come back for a little more later. Above all, don't stretch the skin to the limit by insisting on huge implants.

We can also now increase your breast size without invasive surgery by using fat injections – an incredibly exciting advance.

We would point out that, while breast augmentation can have wonderful results, no surgeon can promise perfection. The best candidates for this procedure, in our opinion, are women who are physically healthy and very realistic in their expectations.

FACTFILE: BREAST AUGMENTATION

- Other names: Breast enlargement, 'boob job'.

- What does it do? Enhances the size and shape of a woman's breasts using implants.

- Type of anaesthetic? General.

- Length of stay? Usually overnight or day care.

- What happens? There are various methods of inserting and positioning implants. The most usual is to make an incision in the crease under the breast. Alternatively the incision can be made in the armpit or around the areola (the darker skin around the nipple). Working through the incision, the surgeon will lift the breast tissue and skin to create a pocket, either directly behind the breast tissue or underneath the pectoral muscle. The chosen implant will then be put into place and centred beneath the nipples. Drains may be used, depending on the position of the implant, the amount of bleeding and whether additional surgery has been carried out. Slow-dissolving stitches or skin glue are used to close the incisions. Your breasts will usually be taped up for further support.

- How does it feel? After surgery you will feel sore, tired and bruised. Many women experience a burning sensation in the nipples or breasts (this usually subsides after a few days).

- How long does it take? One to two hours.

- Scars? Scarring is usually minimal and discreet. However in some women the scars may be red, thick or painful and take several years before improvement.

- Swelling and bruising? At first there will be swelling, hardness and discomfort. Bruising, twinges and pains may continue for the first few weeks.

- Recovery time? You should allow two to three weeks for full recovery, but many women go back to work after a few days.

- Side effects? Capsular (scar) contracture; rupture (a split or hole in the shell of the implant, causing the implant material to leak); seroma (fluid build-up around the implant), rippling and loss of sensation on the nipple for a few months. The usual potential risks of surgery.

- Contraindications? General. Breastfeeding.

- When will I see results? Best results after two months.

- What's the optimum age to have this? Twenties to forties.

- Any other procedures to have at the same time? Breast lifting.

- How long will the results last? Around ten to seventeen years.

- Cost? High.

We say: It's a great operation and very rewarding for both the patient and the surgeon as the results can be so remarkable. But do keep a natural look – a good breast must always look natural. Please don't go to the limit.

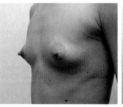 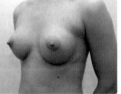

Before   *After*

Breast implants FAQ

Q: What is capsular contracture?

A: This is the most common complication with breast implants (although implants with a textured silicone shell have a lower incidence). The body's natural reaction to any implanted foreign material is to build up scar tissue around it. Scar tissue then shrinks and this shrinkage (known as capsular contracture) can sometimes be noticed as a hardening of the breast. The degree of contracture can vary from person to person, and even from breast to breast. About one in ten women suffer this, and if it happens the implant has to be removed and, if appropriate, replaced with another implant.

Q: What if my implant ruptures?

A: Rupture (a split or hole in the shell of the implant) was common in the early, thin-walled implants. Modern implants are much less likely to do this. Even if the implant does rupture, it does not necessarily cause a medical problem. Saline will be absorbed into the body and naturally excreted. In the majority of cases of silicone implants, the silicone gel will remain within the capsule that the body forms, and will come out alongside the ruptured implant. Occasionally silicone gel may spread outside the capsule into the breast (or, very rarely, into the muscles under the breast, the armpit or the nerves to the arm) where it can create a series of lumps known as siliconomas. These can cause tenderness. In these cases, some breast tissue may be lost when the implant is removed. However if the new high-cohesivity gel is used any leakage is minimal.

Q: Will my new breasts look and feel like 'normal' breasts?

A: Although for most women the implant will feel much like a normal breast, it may be impossible to produce a natural cleavage. Implants may not drop to the side when you lie down and the breasts may feel firmer than normal breast tissue. Creasing, kinking, rippling and folds are possible, particularly in women with very little natural breast tissue.

Q: I've heard I could lose sensations in my nipples. Is this true?

A: About one in seven women report a loss of, or diminished, nipple sensation. On the other hand, some women report nipple sensation is increased for between three to six months following surgery, and this may be uncomfortable.

Q: Will my breasts explode if I fly in an airplane?

A: No, it's a myth. Breast implants are neither strained nor prone to rupture when flying.

Q: Will I be able to breast-feed if I have implants?

A: Yes. Implants do not interfere with the ability to breastfeed although there is some evidence that you might produce slightly less milk. If you have breastfed a baby within the year before your surgery, you may produce milk for a few days following surgery. This may cause some discomfort, but can be treated with medication.

Q: Will having implants increase my risk of breast cancer?

A: No. In fact, the risk may be less (or, at least, the likelihood of a good outcome is better as your breasts will be more carefully monitored and any abnormalities picked up very early). There is no difference between the rate of breast cancer developing or the risk of its recurrence or in survival rates between women with implants and those without.

Q: Will implants interfere with a mammography?

A: It's possible. You should always tell your radiographer that you have implants so they can pick an appropriate method of screening. Be sure to go to a radiology centre where the technicians are experienced in the special techniques required to obtain a reliable X-ray of a breast with an implant. Ultrasound examinations may be of benefit in some women with implants to detect breast lumps or to evaluate the implant.

Q: Do I still need to check my breasts if I have implants?

A: Absolutely. Get to know what is normal for your new breasts and check for changes on a regular basis.

Q: It all sounds so gory. Aren't there less invasive options?

A: Yes. Surgeons are experimenting with using the filler hyaluronic acid. This is injected into the breast to boost breast size. However it would only be temporary, lasting about two years. Even more exciting is the news that fat injection for increasing breast size has very recently been sanctioned. It's a great step forward for less invasive breast augmentation. See page 188 for more information.

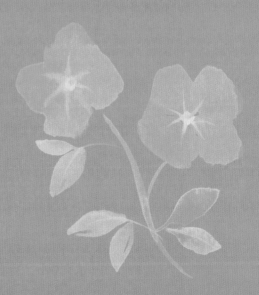

Which implant is best – and safest?

Permanent breast implants are always synthetic or at least they have been until this year and the exciting development of fat injection. Up until now, though, the technique has not been good enough to give permanent results and consequently we have had to use synthetic implants. All synthetic breast implants have a firm elastic shell made of silicone elastomer. The surface of the implant can be either smooth or textured. Inside this shell is the filler, in the UK you will be offered either silicone gel or saline. Both types of filler have been used for a long time and deemed safe. The general life expectancy of all implants is around fifteen years.

There have been a lot of scare stories in the media about the safety of silicone. This has centred around the fact that minute quantities of silicone can diffuse, or 'bleed' through the silicone casing of the implant. It has been suggested that this silicone can cause breast cancer, abnormalities in babies and a range of auto-immune diseases related to arthritis. However, large studies in the US and Europe have proved that there is no increased risk of these diseases in women with breast implants. An independent review by the MHRA on behalf of the Department of Health has concluded that silicone is totally safe, with no evidence of a link with auto-immune disease or cancer. It's also worth pointing out that silicone is frequently used in the body in many other ways, such as wrapping around cardiac pacemakers, with no ill-effects. We therefore feel comfortable using it for cosmetic reasons and tend to prefer it. However many other surgeons use saline with very good results. Let's take a look at the advantages and disadvantages of both.

Silicone gel: implants are filled with either a soft or firm (cohesive) silicone substance. Soft implants are filled with a quite fluid gel while cohesive gel implants contain a more solid, jelly-like gel (we prefer the latest high-cohesivity gel as it minimises the risk of leaking and rupture).

Advantages: less prone to wrinkling and tends to feel much more natural than other implants.

Disadvantages: firm cohesive gels may require a slightly larger scar than those implants using either a saline or soft silicone filler.

Saline: implants are filled with a salt and water solution of a similar concentration to that found in your natural body tissue. Implants are either inserted already filled with the solution, or can be filled through a valve at the time of surgery.

Advantages: the filler is totally natural and, in case of rupture, can be easily absorbed and excreted by the body.

Disadvantages: they may rupture or deflate at an earlier stage than other implants. They are more prone to wrinkling. They tend to look less natural than silicone implants. They don't work so well on women who have little breast tissue.

Implants to avoid

- Soya bean oil-filled implants (Trilucent) are no longer available and the MHRA advises any women with these implants to have them removed.

- Hydrogel implants are also no longer available. They are being monitored by the MHRA but removal is not recommended unless you are experiencing problems with them.

- The shell of some implants can be coated with titanium. These should not be available in the UK and should not be used.

- The shell of some silicone gel implants is coated with a polyurethane foam that breaks down over time. These coated implants were removed from the market in 1991 (over concerns about increased cancer risks) but reintroduced to the UK in 2005. Check the MHRA website (see the Resources section) for detailed information and reports on this type of implant.

NOTE: the MHRA monitors breast implants very carefully. If you have any problems with breast implants you are asked to report them to the organisation (see Resources). The MHRA website also gives very good clear information on implants in general.

CASE STUDY

Alison Lockwood, thirty-one, is a computer analyst from Dublin.

I've always been flat-chested and always felt self-conscious about it. It's bothered me since before I can remember. I've tried every padded bra going and wrestled with pads. I have always felt very insecure about the way I look plus I was truly fed up of not being able to wear what I wanted. I just wanted to look and feel normal.

I put off doing anything about it for years as I was terribly nervous about surgery. But then my best friend had her breasts done and was so ecstatic with the results, I felt I was being ridiculous. I started researching and was very thorough. I visited four surgeons in the end before making my choice. I decided I'd go to a C cup (I had been a AA before); it was quite a jump but I did want to be able to really notice the difference.

I confess I was truly terrified before the op but it was so easy. I honestly had no pain afterwards; I wasn't even groggy (though my friend did say she had a fair amount of pain so maybe I have a high pain threshold). You get great pain medication anyhow and providing you take it correctly I think it's fine. I took arnica too and think that helped me heal swiftly.

I took a week off work and then went in wearing a tight top. I couldn't resist it. I also had my hair cut and I could see people trying to work out if it was just the hair that was different. I was upfront about what I'd done – and about four of my colleagues said I had convinced them to have it done too.

I'd say, to be honest, it was a couple of months before the implants really settled down and I felt completely normal – but I'd been told what to expect and so I wasn't worried at any point. The first time I wore a bikini on the beach was like Christmas and my birthday all rolled into one. I just felt so womanly, so sexy, so normal. My husband, needless to say, loves my new breasts too.

Fat injection: the brand-new real alternative to implants

In the past, if you wanted larger breasts, you had no choice but to have major surgery and implants. Now, at last, there is a real alternative that is safe, effective and only minimally invasive. Fat injection.

It seems so obvious. How many women will ruefully wish they could have a little less down below and a little more up top? If only you could simply suck out a bit of oversized bottom and squirt it into undersized breasts. No invasive surgery, no foreign implants …

While fat injection seemed appealing, it has effectively been forbidden for the last fifteen years – for two major reasons. First it was deemed dangerous: there were concerns that fat could mask the signs of possible breast cancer, or give false readings on mammographs. Second, surgeons simply weren't happy with the results: too much fat was absorbed back into the body.

However the latest thinking turns this on its head. New techniques now mean that fat injections to the breasts are a real – and appealing – option. In America cosmetic surgeons are finding that the new fat injections have a 90 per cent fat survival rate. Up to 300cc of fat can be injected into the breast, taking most breasts up one whole cup size. It's a very safe procedure and the results are nice and natural.

An MRI scan is performed before the procedure, to check that there is no abnormal breast tissue. We then create a pocket in the breast and wait for one month, so the body can create new blood vessels. Then the fat is injected on top of the breast tissue. A further MRI scan is carried out six months after surgery. The beauty of this is that patients can see, quite clearly, the increase in fatty tissue. MRI scans take away the concerns of misleading mammographs.

We are very excited about this new development and are confident that, providing the new guidelines are followed, it is an extremely safe, effective procedure. We shall certainly be introducing it into our own practice.

FACTFILE: BREAST LIFT

- Other names: Mastoplexy.

- What does it do? Raises the breast tissue, repositions the nipple and generally enhances the shape of the breast, making it more pert and youthful. It is specifically for women suffering from drooping or sagging breasts, or stretched nipples. Many women have it after losing a lot of weight or after breastfeeding children. NOTE: it does not increase the size of the breast.

- Type of anaesthetic? General or sedation.

- Length of stay? Overnight.

- What happens? There are three major methods for lifting the breasts. The first is used mainly for larger breasts and involves two incisions in the shape of an anchor – one underneath the breast, and one from the nipple to under the breast. Excess skin is removed, the nipple is moved up and the skin around the nipple is pulled tightly to reshape the breast. The second is usually used for smaller breasts and is known as the 'doughnut': it involves one circular incision around the areola of the nipple (technically known as a periareolar or circumareola) and a doughnut-shaped chunk of tissue is removed. The third involves a periareolar together with a single vertical incision from the areola to the bottom of the breast.

- How does it feel? Expect your breasts to feel very sore and tender for a week or so.

- How long does it take? An hour and a half to three hours.

- Scars? Yes, but surgery is designed to minimise scarring and generally only faint lines can be seen.

- Swelling and bruising? Yes, a lot. Expect your breasts to be bruised, swollen and sore for several weeks.

- Recovery time? Stitches are removed one to two weeks following surgery and you should expect to take that amount of time off work. You will have to wear a support bra (day and night) for up to a month following surgery.

- Side effects? Breasts may stay red and lumpy for some months. Normal risk factors for all surgery. Very rarely unevenly positioned nipples, permanent loss of feeling in nipples or breasts.

- Contraindications? General, breastfeeding.

- When will I see results? About a month following surgery.

- What's the optimum age to have this? Thirties upwards.

- Any other procedures to have at the same time? Breast enlargement.

- How long will the results last? It varies enormously. Larger breasts will sag again more swiftly. As a rule of thumb, about ten years or more.

- Cost? High.

We say: A good effective procedure. We usually prefer to perform the vertical lift so scarring is less noticeable.

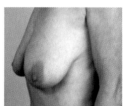 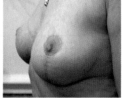

Before　　　　　*After*

FACTFILE: BREAST REDUCTION

- Other names: Reduction mammoplasty.

- What does it do? The breasts are remodelled by removing excess tissue and carefully reshaping the breasts. Size and weight are reduced and shape can be improved.

- Type of anaesthetic? General.

- Length of stay? Usually overnight in hospital.

- What happens? As with breast lifting, there are various methods of breast reduction. The most common is the 'anchor' method, cutting around the areola, down from the areola to under the breast, and then under the natural crease of the breast. Excess tissue and skin are removed. The nipple and areola are moved to a higher position and skin from the sides of the breast is pulled down and around the areola to make a smaller, tighter, firmer shape. Or a vertical incision may be used. Liposuction or LipoSelection is often used to remove excess fat in the breast and armpit area. Drains are inserted if necessary and the wounds are closed up and the breasts bandaged.

- How does it feel? Expect your breasts to feel very sore and tender for several weeks following surgery.

- How long does it take? Between two and four hours.

- Scars? Yes, you must be aware that permanent scarring is inevitable and, because of the nature of the operation, will be far more noticeable than in most other surgery. You should expect lumpy red scars for several months but these will gradually fade and become less obvious over time.

- Swelling and bruising? Yes, swelling can last for several weeks.

- Recovery time? You could be off work for about two weeks. Stitches are removed after one to two weeks and you will need to wear a support bra continually for up to a month. You should expect some tenderness and swelling for several weeks.

- Side effects? Possible complications include loss of sensation in the nipple, inability to breastfeed, lopsided nipples. Plus the usual risks associated with surgery. Asymmetry.

- Contraindications? General, breastfeeding. If you are prone to keloid scars you should be aware that scars could be raised and very visible.

- When will I see results? Optimum results after a couple of months.

- What's the optimum age to have this? Any time after the breasts have fully developed (i.e. over twenty).

- Any other procedures to have at the same time? Liposuction or LipoSelection.

- How long will the results last? Results are permanent, unless you gain excess weight.

  Cost? High.

We say: A very effective procedure that can improve quality of life hugely for many women. Bear in mind, however, that this really is major surgery.

Breast lifting/reduction:FAQ

Q: Will I still be able to breastfeed following a breast lift, or breast reduction?

A: Technically yes after a breast lift, as the milk ducts and nipples are not touched during the procedure. There is more risk of losing the ability to breastfeed following breast reduction. To be entirely safe, we recommend our patients wait until they have completed their family before having either form of surgery.

Q: I've heard it's common to lose feeling in your nipples. Is this correct?

A: It's not common, but it is possible. Again, it's far more likely with a breast reduction than a breast lift, but it is a potential side effect of both procedures.

Q: I hate the idea of such invasive surgery. Are there any other options available?

A: Surgeons are experimenting with botulinum to lift sagging breasts (but it would only work on smaller breasts). It is possible to reduce the size and weight of breasts using LipoSelection but this will only work if the breast is mainly made up of fatty tissue (see below).

Q: I've heard horror stories of nipples dropping off – is this true?

A: In extremely rare cases, yes, the nipple tissue will be rejected.

LipoSelection: the alternative to breast reduction

This is now a very real option for women with large breasts who are uneasy about the major surgery involved with breast reduction. It is particularly suited to women whose breasts have good skin quality, good nipple position and which are mostly fatty tissue. It's also ideal for evening out a breast that is larger than the other, and can be used following a traditional breast reduction if further weight needs to be removed. Generally speaking, the younger you are the better the results, as skin tone will be good and gravity will not have had the chance to set in quite so dramatically – late teens and twenties are ideal. However it still remains an attractive proposition for older women who are willing to trade the lifting and reshaping benefits of traditional surgery with tiny scars, less bruising and swelling, quicker recovery and fewer side effects. Another large plus factor for fat removal is that, in most cases, nipple sensitivity and the ability to breastfeed are not affected. Another good reason for younger women who have not yet had their families to consider it.

ARMS

Hit forty and, unless you work out like Madonna, it's nigh-on impossible to avoid the dreaded bat wings. Yes, you can certainly disguise them with long sleeves and wraps, but it's a bit limiting. Having surgery on your arms might seem an unlikely idea but it's becoming increasingly popular as a straightforward, swift way to beat the bat.

FACTFILE: ARM LIFT

- Other names: Brachioplasty.

- What does it do? Removes excess fat and skin from the upper arms, giving a firmer, tauter look.

- Type of anaesthetic? General.

- Length of stay? Usually overnight.

- What happens? Long incisions are made along the underside of the upper arm, from the armpit curving down to the elbow. Excess fat and skin is removed. Liposuction may be needed to remove large amounts of fat. The remaining tissue and skin are lifted to create a smoother, tauter profile.

- How does it feel? Expect discomfort and tightness, also numbness is possible for up to several months.

- How long does it take? About two hours.

- Scars? Yes, you will have long fine scars stretching from the armpit to the elbow.

- Swelling and bruising? Yes, swelling in particular is quite severe and can last for several months.

- Recovery time? Expect to be off work for one to two weeks. You won't be able to exercise for four to six weeks.

- Side effects? A lop-sided appearance is possible but very rare. The usual complications of surgery are possible but rare.

- Contraindications? People prone to infections in the sweat gland; people who have had mastectomy, following operations in the axilla lymph node.

- When will I see results? When the swelling subsides, after a few months.

- What's the optimum age to have this? Any age, but usually after forty, or following dramatic weight loss.

- Any other procedures to have at the same time? LipoSelection.

- How long will the results last? Permanently, providing you do not put on weight.

- Cost? High.

We say: It's an expensive invasive procedure. LipoSelection may provide a good alternative that is far less invasive – and far cheaper.

FAT REMOVAL

Virtually everyone has got some – a bit of fat that simply won't do the decent thing and disappear. Whether it's on your bottom, your thighs, your tummy or your knees, there is a simple, highly effective answer: liposuction. Well, we say liposuction, but truly there are now far better, less invasive forms than the original fat hoovering of liposuction. The original liposuction is pretty invasive – it damages a lot of tissue other than fat and often you will see nearly as much blood as fat being removed. Then ultrasound came along and we were able to be far more selective about what was removed. Ultrasound liposuction is able to differentiate between fat and body tissue that really shouldn't be extracted (such as blood vessels, nerves and connective tissue). The result is that the ratio of fat to blood being extracted rose exponentially.

However now technology has moved on again. LipoSelection is the newest treatment, truly the 'next generation' of ultrasound liposuction. It is an incredibly gentle technique and the most advanced approach to fat removal available at present; in fact the technology is so gentle and specific that it was originally designed to treat brain tumours.

It gently and precisely reshapes the body by the removal of fat pockets. What makes LipoSelection different is that it can target body fat even more effectively by the use of a special saline solution that liquefies the fat cells before removal. This causes far less trauma and the skin can retract smoothly and evenly after the procedure, minimising the pain and bruising typically associated with fat removal, so most patients experience a fast recovery and return to normal activities within days.

We would thoroughly recommend you find a clinic that uses LipoSelection if you possibly can. If not, then do ensure you at least have ultrasound liposuction (often called Liposculpture) as it is far less invasive than standard liposuction.

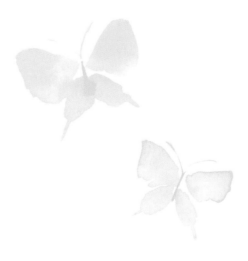

FACTFILE: LIPOSELECTION

- What does it do? Takes away excess fatty tissue by dissolving fat cells and then extracting them.

- Type of anaesthetic? Local anaesthetic with sedation.

- Length of stay? Two hours following surgery.

- What happens? The area to be sculpted is filled with a special saline solution and local anaesthetic that helps to numb the site and shrink the blood vessels (to minimise blood loss and bruising). It also makes the fat cells easier to liquefy. Then small probes are inserted which transmit sound energy: this targets and dissolves fat cells while harmlessly bouncing off other tissue. The emulsified fat flows into the saline solution and is easily extracted in liquid form.

- How does it feel? There is some soreness and tenderness afterwards.

- How long does it take? Between one and four hours, depending on how much fat is removed.

- Scars? Absolutely minimal.

- Swelling and bruising? Yes, but far less than with normal liposuction.

- Recovery time? Forty-eight hours to recover from the anaesthetic. You will need to wear a special garment twenty-four hours a day for one week, and will not be able to shower during this time. You return after a week to have your bandages and stitches removed. However (within these restrictions) you can return to work within days and be back to the gym after one week.

- Side effects? The usual risks associated with all surgery apply. Other risks are unlikely but could include contour irregularities, prolonged swelling or numbing, blister-like spots (seromas), burns, skin discolouration.

- Contraindications? General.

- When will I see results? Four weeks after surgery.

- What's the optimum age to have this? Any.

- Any other procedures to have at the same time? We recommend a course of Endermologie before and after LipoSelection.

- How long will the results last? Results are permanent, providing you do not put on more weight.

- Cost? Medium – high.

We say: This is a truly exciting new and gentle technology. We recommend it to all our patients as the results are excellent and it causes far less stress and trauma to the body.

COMPARING FAT REMOVAL TECHNIQUES

TYPE OF FAT REMOVAL	LIPOSUCTION	LIPOSCULPTURE	LIPOSELECTION
Type of anaesthetic	General	Local with IV sedation	Local with IV sedation
Length of stay	One day	Day care	Two hours following surgery
Back to work	One week	One week	Within two days
Other considerations	More bruising, swelling and pain	Useful for evening out previous skin deformities by removing fat and re-injecting it elsewhere	Less traumatic and quicker recovery time, a far smoother result

Fat removal: FAQ

Q: How much fat can be removed?

A: There are limits. A certain amount of body fat is vital for good health. Also, the deepest layers of fat (those surrounding and protecting your vital organs) cannot be taken safely. Let your surgeon advise you on how much fat it is safe to remove. If you are a day care patient (with local/IV sedation), the maximum is 4 litres. If you have a general anaesthetic you can go further but you must recognise that this is major surgery and carries more risks. For safety we prefer to do major LipoSelection in two stages. It is less risky, less painful and has much better results.

Q: Does fat removal take away the entire fat cell – or just the fat in it?

A: It takes away the entire cell. However, because fat is necessary to a healthy body, some essential fat will remain untreated in any area.

Q: Can the fat grow back?

A: Once you have fat removed, it's gone and, assuming you keep up a healthy lifestyle of proper diet and exercise, it won't return or migrate to other areas. However, if you do gain a lot of weight, the remaining fat cells will expand and you will look fatter.

Q: I need to lose a lot of weight – can't it just all be sucked away?

A: Sadly not. No form of liposuction is a real weight loss solution. If you have a lot of weight to lose, the best solution is a combination of sensible diet and exercise (see the Natural Rejuvenation Plan).

Q: Will liposuction sort out my cellulite?

A: Sorry, but it's very unlikely. You may notice an improvement in the appearance of your cellulite, but it's unrealistic to expect any form of liposuction to eliminate or 'fix' cellulite. There is no surgical procedure that can do that.

CASE STUDY

Georgia Davidson, twenty-nine, is a marketing consultant from Swansea.

I'm fit and healthy and I go to the gym regularly. I eat a good diet but no matter what I did I simply couldn't get rid of my love handles or a thickness on my thighs. I was conscious of it in my jeans and it really bothered me. When I saw Maurizio he said that, sadly, lipo was the only thing that would really change my shape so I made up my mind to do it. We decided to target my inner and outer thighs, plus the dreaded love handles.

I was absolutely petrified about the idea of surgery because I'd never had anything done to me before. In fact I was so focused on the operation itself it never dawned on me to think it might be painful or uncomfortable afterwards! My anaesthetist was absolutely lovely though and I don't remember a thing about the operation. When I woke up I was in the recovery room, all snuggled up in a warm-air blanket. I felt absolutely fine, though very cold (this is common with sedation). I had something to eat and then went home. I felt tired but that was it.

When I looked at my legs, though, I had quite a shock – they were totally black and blue. I was so bruised. It was also a bit uncomfortable if I turned over in bed or when I sat down – my thighs were the most tender. I did have a few moments when I thought, Oh heck, what have I done? particularly as they seemed much heavier than before. But by the fourth or fifth week the swelling suddenly just dropped away over the space of a few days.

I was truly delighted with the end result: I no longer have that wodge of flab hanging over my low-rise jeans and my thighs look gorgeous. I'm also totally over my fear of operations – I'm planning a nose job next!

THE STOMACH

It's a tough fact that, while fashion dictates a flat, even concave stomach, nature provides most women with a rounded belly. If that is your only problem, we'd suggest you look at diet (wheat intolerance can often cause a bloated stomach), deep core toning exercises or possibly a little LipoSelection. However, as women get older, and particularly when they have children, the entire tummy area can often require a bit more help. We have seen countless women come to us in desperation because their stomachs have, quite literally, gone south. They no longer feel able to wear their favourite clothes, and the idea of braving the beach in a bikini is too horrible to contemplate.

It's not usually a question of being overweight. What often happens is that a woman is left (often after pregnancy and particularly following Caesareans) with a flabby abdomen, or an 'apron' of skin that hangs down in a deep fold. At this stage, we think in terms of a tummy tuck. A tummy tuck is a major surgical procedure to remove excess skin and fat from the middle and lower abdomen, and to tighten the muscles of the abdominal wall. It is a big operation but the results can be quite dramatic, reducing the appearance of a protruding abdomen and creating a smoother, flatter tummy. The overall results will, however, depend very much on your skin tone, how old you are and how much weight you are carrying. We often advise patients who are overweight to diet before undertaking this surgery. LipoSelection on the abdomen can take away any remaining excess fat.

Before you decide upon any abdominal surgery it's vital that you consult an experienced surgeon. If your fat deposits are limited to the area below the navel, you may require a far less complex procedure, the mini tummy tuck. If your hips and buttocks are the major problem a lower belt lift might be more suitable. If you do not have too much lax skin, LipoSelection alone may be possible. On the other hand, you might require a combination of a tummy tuck with LipoSelection to smooth the contours of your hips as well as your abdomen.

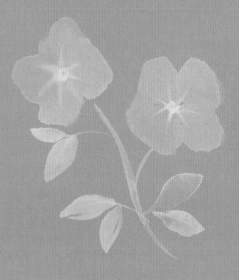

FACTFILE: TUMMY TUCK

- Other names: Abdominoplasty.

- What does it do? Removes excess fat and skin from the entire abdominal area (both above and below the navel). Tightens abdominal muscles. Slims down and tones sagging, bulging stomachs.

- Type of anaesthetic? General.

- Length of stay? Usually overnight.

- What happens? A large incision is made from hip-bone to hip-bone across the abdomen, just over the pubic bone. Another incision separates the navel from the surrounding tissue. The skin is separated from the abdominal wall and fat deposits are removed. The muscles are pulled, tightened and then stitched into position, providing a stronger abdominal wall. Excess skin is removed and the skin is pulled down and stitched up. A new hole is incised for the navel which is then stitched back into its new position.

- How does it feel? You should expect a degree of discomfort, and strenuous activity must be avoided for three to four weeks.

- How long does it take? It depends how much fat needs to be removed. Between two and five hours.

- Scars? Yes, there is a permanent scar across the abdomen, but it is low-lying and usually hidden by underwear.

- Swelling and bruising? Yes, considerable swelling in particular, which may last for several months.

- Recovery time? This is a serious procedure and you should not expect to be back to your usual lifestyle for about a month to six weeks. How long you take off work will depend on the nature of your work, but bear in mind that standing up straight will cause discomfort (most people are able to return after two to four weeks). You will need to wear a support garment for about a month. Stitches are removed after about two weeks.

- Side effects? Many people find their abdomen feels numb for some months. An irregular or lopsided appearance is possible but rare. The usual rare complications for surgery apply. A seroma (an accumulation of serum – rather like a non-infectious abscess) is possible.

- Contraindications? General. Also, this is not suitable if you plan to become pregnant in the future.

- When will I see results? When the swelling subsides, after a few months.

- What's the optimum age to have this? Any age, but really only after you have completed your family. It is particularly suitable for women whose skin and muscle have been stretched by pregnancy, or who have lost considerable amounts of weight, leaving loose and overhanging skin and flab.

- Any other procedures to have at the same time? Lipsuction, LipoSelection but in different areas (not the abdomen).

- How long will the results last? Permanently, providing you do not put on weight.

- Cost? High.

We say: This can dramatically reduce the appearance of a protruding abdomen, and is particularly helpful for women who, through multiple pregnancies, have stretched abdominal skin and muscles. It is a good, effective procedure but it is major surgery. We would also point out that, if you are very overweight, you should lose weight before you have surgery. Also, we don't recommend it if you are planning future pregnancies.

CASE STUDY

Joanna Webb-Green, forty-six, is a hairdresser from Somerset.

I'd had it up to here with my body. I would have to say I've never been totally happy with it but once I had my three children it just became completely out of control. I had a huge roll of flab that wouldn't shift no matter how much weight I lost. It just hung over my waistband – not a good look. Going to the gym was really embarrassing – I was the only one wearing a vast sweatshirt to cover up the flab. It took me quite a while to decide to have it done but, once I'd made up my mind, I just couldn't wait.

My husband was great about it. The operation isn't cheap and you have to take a fair bit of time off work (and can't do any lifting or heavy work so housework was out!). But he really supported me all the way, and I would say it's really essential to have a high level of support at home if you're considering this operation. I was dreading telling my mother but she surprised me by being all for it, in fact she said she wished she had the nerve to do it herself.

It was painful, I must be honest. When I came to it felt as if someone were raking my stomach. But the painkillers are good and I just kept focusing on the end result. Having a drain was weird though. I hadn't expected to see what seemed like a lot of fluid coming out, but I was reassured it was totally normal. I seemed to sleep most of the time for the first few days, and after a week I felt like a totally different person. You have to be patient with this operation – don't expect instant results. At first I thought it was a complete disaster. I just couldn't notice any difference and I felt like an idiot, that I'd wasted all that time and money and put myself through major surgery for nothing. I'd been told, time and time again, that the swelling would make it impossible to notice anything at first but I just didn't take it in. However when I was finally able to take off the support garment I realised what a difference it had made. I actually had a real woman's shape again, I wasn't a bag lady any more.

A tummy tuck is a big commitment and a major operation, but I felt it was totally worth every penny and every bit of discomfort. It's as if my body and I have made friends again – and that's a much more comfortable way to be.

FACTFILE: MINI-TUMMY TUCK

- Other names: Partial abdominoplasty.

- What does it do? Removes excess fat and sagging skin from the stomach (below the navel) to create a flatter, tauter stomach. This is a less invasive procedure than a full tummy tuck as the navel will not require repositioning.

- Type of anaesthetic? General or epidural combined with IV sedation.

- Length of stay? Usually overnight.

- What happens? A large incision is made running across the lower abdomen, just above your pubic bone. The skin is lifted, fat is removed and any excess skin is removed. Liposuction may be required. Then the skin is stretched back down and stitched.

- How does it feel? Expect pain for a few days following surgery. Your stomach will feel tight and very swollen. Many people experience a tugging feeling when they try to stand up straight. Numbness in the abdominal area is also quite common and this can last for several months.

- How long does it take? About one to two hours.

- Scars? Yes, there is a long permanent scar stretching from hip to hip across the abdomen.

- Swelling and bruising? Yes, swelling in particular is substantial and may last for several months.

- Recovery time? Expect to be off work for about two weeks, or more.

- Side effects? The usual (rare) complications for surgery.

- Contraindications? General. This procedure is not suitable if you plan to become pregnant in the future.

- When will I see results? When the swelling subsides, after a few weeks.

- What's the optimum age to have this? Any age, but it's best if you are not generally excessively overweight but just hold excess weight in the lower abdominal area.

- Any other procedures to have at the same time? Liposuction or LipoSelection.

- How long will the results last? Permanently, providing you do not put on weight.

- Cost? High.

We say: Well worth considering if your fat deposits are limited to the area below your navel. This is a much less complex procedure than the standard tummy tuck and many women like the fact that the navel is left untouched. It can be combined well with LipoSelection. However, as with the full abdominoplasty, we don't advise you to have this procedure until you have completed your family.

FACTFILE: LOWER BODY LIFT

- Other names: Belt Lipectomy.

- What does it do? Removes excess skin and fat from the lower body – abdomen, hips, lower back. Also lifts the buttocks and thighs. Tautens the underlying muscle of the abdomen.

- Type of anaesthetic? General.

- Length of stay? Up to two days.

- What happens? Incisions are made across the buttocks and on the inner and outer thighs. Crescent-shaped segments of skin and fat are removed from the buttock and thigh areas. Liposuction is usually used to remove excess fat around the hips and lower back. The remaining tissue and skin are then lifted and stitched.

- How does it feel? This is a tough procedure and involves a significant amount of pain and discomfort.

- How long does it take? Around four or five hours (depending on extent of surgery and any liposuction).

- Scars? Yes, you will have long scars across the buttocks and inside and outside your thighs (where possible these are positioned so they will be hidden by underwear).

- Swelling and bruising? Yes, considerable. Swelling may not disappear for three or four months.

- Recovery time? Expect to take at least two weeks off work. You will not be able to exercise for about six weeks.

- Side effects? Rarely the lymphatic system in the groin is affected, causing severe swelling (oedema) for a few weeks. The usual complications of surgery are possible (but rare).

- Contraindications? General. Phlebitis (inflammation of veins).

- When will I see results? When the swelling subsides, after a few months.

- What's the optimum age to have this? This is mainly suited to people who have lost a considerable amount of weight, leaving them with large amounts of sagging skin.

- Any other procedures to have at the same time? Tummy tuck, LipoSelection.

- How long will the results last? Permanently, providing you do not put on weight.

- Cost? High.

We say: This is very invasive major surgery. Think carefully. It is a valid operation for certain patients but it is a very specific procedure and there can be a lot of complications. Pick a surgeon with a great deal of experience in this particular field of cosmetic surgery (known as bariatric surgery).

THE BUTTOCKS

Nowadays the question often isn't 'Does my bum look big in this?' but 'Does my bum look too small?' Firm, well-rounded buttocks are incredibly fashionable nowadays, with celebrities like J-Lo and Beyoncé waving the flag for big-bottomed girls. As we get older, sadly, buttocks start to droop and sag. Some also become overly flabby and fatty. None of these looks great, particularly if you're wearing tight jeans or want to strip off for the beach. Excess flab can easily be removed using liposuction or LipoSelection. However for the best possible shape you may well need a little more help in the shape of a buttock lift or the use of implants (silicone implants are most usual).

We must warn you that buttock surgery can involve a fair amount of discomfort; if you think about it, we use our buttocks all the time – even when we are sitting down or sleeping – so it's impossible to avoid a certain amount of tenderness.

FACTFILE: BUTTOCK LIFT

- What does it do? Tightens and lifts sagging, drooping buttocks giving a younger, perter look.

- Type of anaesthetic? General.

- Length of stay? Usually overnight.

- What happens? Semicircular-shaped segments of skin and fat are removed from the buttocks and the remaining skin and tissue is lifted to create the new tighter, firmer shape. Excess fat can be taken out with LipoSelection.

- How does it feel? Afterwards you will feel very sore and sitting will be uncomfortable. You may also experience numbness (which may last for a few months).

- How long does it take? One to two hours.

- Scars? Yes, the scar can be quite long and stretches straight across the buttocks where it is visible. However it is usually hidden by underwear.

- Swelling and bruising? Yes, light bruising and considerable swelling (which may last up to four months).

- Recovery time? You'll need to take a week off work. You will need to wear a support garment for a month to help with reshaping.

- Side effects? Very rarely you can experience a lopsided or irregular appearance to the buttocks. The usual complications for any form of surgery apply.

- Contraindications? Patients who have had phlebitis in their legs may not be suitable candidates for this surgery.

- When will I see results? After the swelling subsides, after about four months typically.

- What's the optimum age to have this? Any age, but usually thirty plus.

- Any other procedures to have at the same time? Liposuction or LipoSelection.

- How long will the results last? Permanent, unless you gain a lot of weight.

- Cost? High.

We say: We are not very happy with this procedure at the moment as scarring is very noticeable. In the future, however, there may well be alternatives. Research is going on at the moment in South America and Korea looking at thread lifts for the buttocks. Our advice is wait and see what comes next.

FACTFILE: BUTTOCK AUGMENTATION

- Other names: Buttock implants.

- What does it do? Reshapes a flat or unsightly bottom, producing a more rounded pleasing shape.

- Type of anaesthetic? General.

- Length of stay? Usually overnight.

- What happens? A two- to three- inch incision is made between the buttocks. The muscle is lifted up and a pocket is made for the implant (ensuring that both sides match perfectly). The implants are inserted and secured.

- How does it feel? Expect to feel very sore. You may also experience some numbness around the buttocks (which may last for some months).

- How long does it take? About an hour and a half.

- Scars? Yes, but usually hidden in the crease of the buttocks.

- Swelling and bruising? Yes, swelling can be considerable and last for a few months.

- Recovery time? Time off work: two weeks. You will need to wear a support hose for about a month.

- Side effects? The usual (rare) reactions to surgery apply: infection, bleeding, haematoma, nerve damage, bad reaction to anaesthetic. This is a very painful procedure.

- Contraindications? General. Phlebitis. Use of high-dose steroids.

- When will I see results? When the swelling subsides, after a few months.

- What's the optimum age to have this? Any age.

- Any other procedures to have at the same time? LipoSelection.

- How long will the results last? It depends on the filler used – from a year to permanently.

- Cost? High.

We say: Frankly, we would advise a much more natural approach. A good exercise programme can have great results.

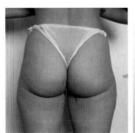

Before

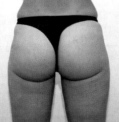

After

THIGHS AND HIPS

'Thunder thighs', 'hamhocks', 'child-bearing hips': a womanly shape is all well and good but thick chunky thighs and broad solid hips are hardly every woman's dream. Fashion is particularly cruel with skinny jeans and body-hugging fabrics clinging to every (excessive) curve – it's no wonder most pear-shapes opt to hide in voluminous skirts. Come summer and you're swathed in sarongs or covered up in kaftans rather than bare your legs. A thigh lift could be the answer as the procedure can take away large amounts of excess flab. However, this is at present not a common procedure – and it is quite extreme. Ensure your surgeon is very experienced with this procedure. You will also need to discuss your overall proportions with your surgeon. If you lose a lot of weight from the upper part of the leg, your lower legs might look out of proportion. Some people find they require work on their calves to balance the look.

FACTFILE: THIGH LIFT

- Other names: Thighplasty.

- What does it do? Removes large amounts of fat and skin from the hips and thighs, giving a much leaner, more toned profile.

- Type of anaesthetic? General.

- Length of stay? Usually overnight.

- What happens? Segments of skin and fat are removed from the thighs and hips. The remaining tissue is lifted to achieve a taut, smooth effect. LipoSelection is frequently used in tandem to remove excess fat.

- How does it feel? This procedure can cause a lot of pain and discomfort following the operation. You may well experience numbness around the thighs for several months following surgery.

- How long does it take? About two to three hours.

- Scars? Yes, there are long scars extending across the outer and inner thighs. Where possible, they will be hidden by the bikini line.

- Swelling and bruising? Yes, considerable bruising and swelling, and the swelling can last for several months.

- Recovery time? You will need to take two weeks off work. You will need to wear a support garment for three to four weeks following surgery.

- Side effects? The lymphatic system in the groin may be affected during surgery, causing considerable swelling (oedema) for a few months. The usual surgical risks apply. Seroma.

- Contraindications? General. Phlebitis.

- When will I see results? When the swelling subsides, after a few months.

- What's the optimum age to have this? Any age. Frequently following extreme weight loss.

- Any other procedures to have at the same time? LipoSelection. Buttock lift.

- How long will the results last? Permanently, providing you do not put on weight.

- Cost? High.

We say: We don't like this procedure as there is too much scarring and the result is not long-lasting. Frankly, it's not one of the best cosmetic procedures. Think about LipoSelection and a great toning programme.

What to do if it goes wrong

First of all, don't panic. Many procedures can be reversed; others can be improved and changed. Implants can be removed – for good or exchanged for something smaller or a different shape. They can also easily be repositioned. Facelifts that are too tight can be repositioned or redraped for a more natural look. Uneven liposuction can be smoothed out with further work. Even nose jobs that are too extreme can be remedied with implants. Possibly the most difficult procedure to fix is one around the eyes, where the skin is particularly delicate and thin, but clever surgeons can do wonders.

However, before you complain, do remember that any change is going to be a shock. Ask yourself honestly if your expectations were reasonable. Ask other people for their honest opinion: has the procedure really gone wrong or been done badly, or do you just need to get used to it?

Have you given your body or face time to recover? Do bear in mind that you often won't see the full effects of your surgery for some days or even weeks or months. Don't judge a procedure halfway through the recovery time; most people go through a period of 'it hasn't worked' or 'it's not what I hoped for' while the bruising and swelling remain.

However, if something really has gone wrong, you will need to take steps.

All clinics and hospitals that are registered with the Healthcare Commission are required to have a policy dealing with complaints.

- Tell the clinic you are unhappy with your treatment. Talk to your surgeon and ask for his advice.

- Discuss the problem and see if it can be resolved. It may be that your healing process is not complete and your body still needs time to heal properly or settle down.

- If you are still unhappy after the full recovery time, and your expectations were not unrealistic, they may offer further treatment or surgery to rectify the problem.

- If you are still unhappy, you should write a formal letter of complaint to your clinic and also make a complaint to the Healthcare Commission or the Independent Healthcare Forum (providing the clinic, hospital or salon is a member). These bodies can take action against a clinic if it is in breach of the standards it is expected to meet. However they cannot deal with complaints relating to fees or with complaints against unregistered practitioners.

- You can also complain to Trading Standards, regardless of whether your clinic is registered or not.

- If your complaint is about the performance or conduct of your surgeon or doctor, you can complain to the General Medical Council.

- If you are not happy allowing your original surgeon to perform remedial work, you should find someone else. Find a surgeon who is skilled at doing secondary revisional procedures. This is a specialty, particularly for tricky revisions such as rhinoplasty and eyelid surgery.

- Bear in mind that you may not be able to have major revisions immediately. Secondary surgery is not usually recommended for between six and twelve months after the original procedure.

CHAPTER NINE

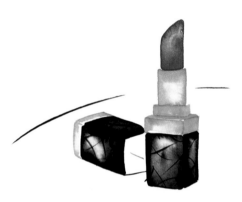

The final touches

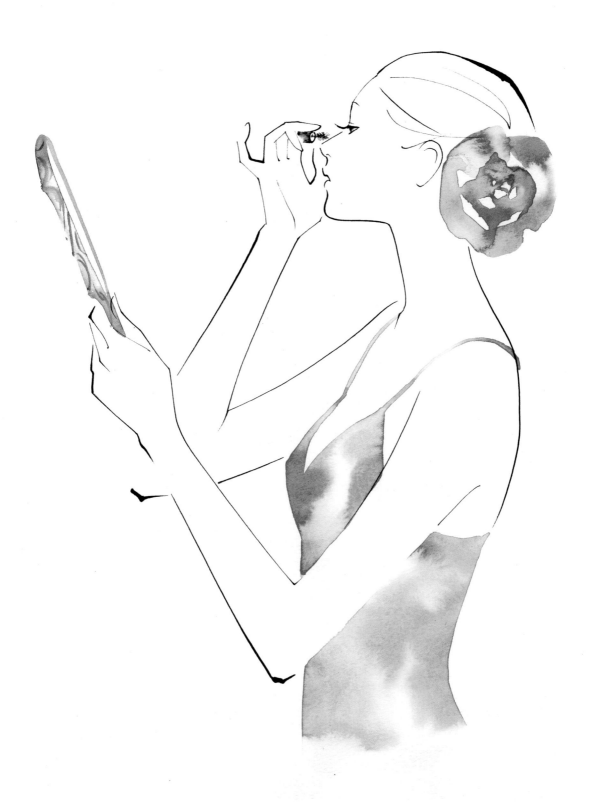

The work isn't finished when you walk out of the clinic. If you want to get the most out of your new look you may need to make just a few more changes. Nothing major – just a tweak here or there. It's a good idea to look at your entire overall look: how you wear your hair, how you use make-up, which clothes you wear. Often a few shifts or twists will be in order to maximise the impact of the new you.

Posture is another vital component. So many of our patients have learned over the years to hide their bodies with poor posture that often we have to insist they relearn how to hold themselves. After all, what's the point of having gorgeous new breasts, for example, if you're going to slump your shoulders and hide them?

You may also find that you not only look different, but you feel quite different emotionally as well. Most people underestimate the psychological effects of cosmetic surgery. They simply aren't prepared for what happens inside when you shift the way you look on the outside.

You've come a long way. Let's just add the finishing touches.

Your new face or body

If you're having a relatively small procedure (such as a filler, a peel or even eyelid surgery) you'll probably adjust to your new look easily and swiftly. When you look in the mirror you'll see a familiar face – simply one that is younger- and fresher-looking. But if you have major surgery, such as breast augmentation or reduction, rhinoplasty, a tummy tuck or facelift, these can involve quite a radical shift in the way you look and may require a longer time of adjustment. When you look in the mirror you will see someone quite different looking back at you, and many people find this disconcerting, even unsettling or unpleasant.

Don't be surprised if this happens. It's completely normal. Also do remember that the vast majority of surgery will leave you looking rather worse before you look better, which is perfectly natural given that your body or face has been through quite a bit of trauma. You will look in the mirror and see a swollen, bruised, rather battered-looking you.

Sometimes, even when the bruising goes, you are left feeling a little let-down, a sort of 'so that's it' feeling. Again, this is quite natural. Most people find they feel slightly low following surgery but this usually passes fairly quickly. However some people do experience post-operative depression. This usually sets in about three days after surgery, as your strength returns but your appearance is still a bit battered. It can last just a few days (most people find it passes within the week) or it can persist for several weeks. There's no precise reason for this depression, but it seems likely it's brought on by a combination of stress, post-surgery tiredness and the lack of immediate visible results. If you're undergoing a procedure that takes place in stages, it's more common to experience depression as you have to deal with an 'unfinished' image for an extended period.

If you do feel depressed following surgery:

- Talk to your surgeon.
- Try taking light exercise (if advised by your surgeon).
- Get out into the fresh air.
- Talk to supportive friends.
- Remind yourself that this is just a phase, it will pass.

On the other hand, you may react quite differently. For some people, the elation of their new image can be equally hard to handle. It's not unknown for people to feel so liberated and free following surgery that their behaviour can be quite erratic and surprising. You might even lose the plot a little, and it's important not to be too hasty when it comes to launching yourself into new relationships or sexual encounters following surgery. Give yourself a little time to adjust to your new image. Take it slow.

Your post-surgery recovery plan
After surgery, follow these essential tips.

1 Follow the guidelines given to you by your clinic or surgeon. Don't try to be smart or think you are the exception to the rule – do what they suggest.

2 Take your homeopathic remedies and, when advised by your surgeon, resume your supplements.

3 Use ice for the first twenty-four to forty-eight hours to cut down on swelling and bruising. It doesn't matter if you use a proper gel mask or a pack of frozen peas, the aim is simply to apply cold to the affected area.

4 Rest as much as possible. Your body has been through a trauma so give it time to recover.

5 Don't fret over whether you have the effect you want at this point. It's not a cut and dried process and you need to have fully healed before you can see the final result.

6 Make sure your diet is as good as possible. Follow the Beauty Diet guidelines to ensure you are getting all the nutrients your body needs.

7 Get back to exercise as soon as you can. Obviously if you have had major surgery, particularly to the abdomen, you will need to wait for around six weeks. But get outside, go walking, try some qi gong.

Support – and lack of support

Cosmetic surgery often involves major surgery. Yet so many people don't ever think about having a support network in place to help after the operation. It's madness really: you wouldn't think about trying to get by on your own after a hysterectomy or a Caesarean, would you? So how come so few people get adequate support following cosmetic procedures?

Your surgery may have been elective, you may have chosen to undergo it, but that doesn't mean you should battle through alone. Even the most independent soul needs physical and emotional support. But choose your support carefully. Pick someone who will be genuinely supportive. Avoid anyone who is critical of your decision to have surgery; the last thing you need is someone pitching in with 'I don't know why you had surgery – you were fine as you were.' Also avoid people who might be shocked, or disgusted by your swelling and stitches. You need to focus on your recovery, not be beset by doubts and anxieties.

Sadly, there will always be people who will feel the need to criticise or comment on your new appearance. You can't avoid it, so you need to be prepared for it.

- Some people will feel threatened by your wonderful new looks.
- Some people may be very judgemental, feeling that cosmetic surgery is vain and frivolous.
- Some people may be horrified that you spent so much money on your appearance.
- Some people may feel affronted that you changed a family or ethnic trait, and accuse you of denying your genetic or social heritage.
- Some people will be jealous, wishing they had the money or the nerve to do the same.

Remember why you chose to have surgery: keep your goal firmly in sight, and let any criticism wash over your head. You may find it helpful to use a very clear statement of why you had the procedure, something like: 'This is something I chose to do, just for myself. I love it.'

Super skincare

Now you have a lovelier face and body, you need to keep it that way. While regular exercise, eating great food and adding in power-supplements will do tons for your skin, you can help it still further by giving it the best possible ingredients topically (in the form of creams, lotions and serums).

We have already given you the basic skincare regime. Now it's time to introduce you to the superstars of the cosmetic world. Hordes of products now tout themselves as 'anti-ageing', 'rejuvenating' and 'cosmeceutical' (cosmetics that have rejuvenating properties). Of course, these are just names, and merely because a product calls itself a cosmeceutical or anti-ageing doesn't mean it can necessarily really deliver the goods. Also, many of the ingredients that really have a profound effect on your skin can only be obtained from doctors or dermatologists. Having said that, there are many ingredients we do feel are worth seeking out.

This is particularly important when you have had cosmetic procedures. Give your new face or body the best possible creams you can. This is why we developed our own small range of creams, using some of the most exciting ingredients available.

THE TOP TWENTY-FIVE MIRACLE INGREDIENTS: WHAT TO LOOK FOR IN YOUR JAR

1 **Aloe vera**: helps soothe inflammation and gives moisture to the skin. You will need to look out for concentrations of 10 per cent or more, otherwise it simply isn't effective.

2 **Alpha-hydroxy** and **beta-hydroxy acids**: mild fruit and milk acids that help exfoliate and promote a smoother, fresher-looking skin.

3 **Alpha-lipoic acid**: a very powerful antioxidant and anti-inflammatory. We like it and use it in our *X115 Face and Body Cream*. There are two forms of lipoic acid – R and S forms. The R form is the most effective wrinkle-reducer (and the presence of the S form seems to reduce its powers) so ideally look out for products that say explicitly R-lipoic acid.

4 **Argireline** (acetyl hexapeptide-3): argireline really is a miracle ingredient, a peptide that acts as a topical alternative to botulinum, creating a numbing effect to help reduce the kind of movement (e.g. frowning) that creates lines. It's been shown to reduce the depths of lines and wrinkles, fade dark circles, deter the degeneration of collagen and elastin and to make skin firmer, fuller and younger-looking. So it's small wonder we use it in our *X117 Eye Cream*.

5 **Calendula**: deeply soothing, nourishing and healing for the skin.

6 **Co-enzyme Q10**: its superb antioxidant powers make this an obvious choice for anti-ageing products. Research shows that regular use of CoQ10 clearly reduces crow's feet. A similar vitamin-like structure is Idebenone; early research indicates it may be just as useful in skincare as its cousin CoQ10 – watch out for this one.

7 **Copper peptides**: compounds of copper and protein that have distinct wound-healing and skin-soothing properties (so potentially very useful following resurfacing treatments). Less research has been carried out on their ability to rejuvenate skin but it seems possible they could rejuvenate skin cells, improving elasticity, firming the skin and reducing fine lines. They appear to be able to stimulate collagen production and reduce the degradation of collagen that contributes to wrinkles. One to watch.

8 **Cytokinins** (furfuryladenine, kinetin, zeatin): plant-derived growth factors that appear to improve fine lines, blotchy skin and wrinkles. Also improve sun-damaged skin. Have been touted as a gentler alternative to Retin A, but more research needs to be done.

9 **DMAE**: touted in the press as a 'facelift in a jar'. We wouldn't go quite that far but it does have wonderful skin-toning properties. It's an antioxidant membrane stabiliser which also gives protection from free radicals. It helps to repair collagen and make skin firmer. We use it in our *X115 Face and Body Cream* because it can quickly and dramatically improve the appearance of saggy skin. It also boosts the effect of other antioxidants, resulting in extra smoothness, brightness and line reduction. We advise all our patients to take it in supplement form too, so the cream is even more effective.

10 **GABA** (gamma-amino-butyric acid): a clever ingredient that makes muscles relax and so gives a softening effect to fine lines and wrinkles.

11 **Green tea extract**: its properties come from flavonoid phytochemicals known as polyphenols (in particular catechins).

Applied topically it can help protect your skin from sun damage (and may boost your sunscreen too). It also appears very useful in lessening wrinkles and boosting skin tone.

12 **Hyaluronic acid** (hyaluron): once again, this wonder-substance comes to the rescue of our skin. Increasingly used in good formulae (not just moisturisers but also cleansers) to help the skin retain moisture and plump it out.

13 **Lipids**: fats that form a natural part of the skin's protective barrier. Natural forms are ceramides, free fatty acids, sphingolipids and sterols. Synthetic forms are usually known as ceramides.

14 **Lycopene**: one of the plant pigments known as carotenes. It's a powerful antioxidant, helps improve cell metabolism and can help protect your skin from sun damage. It's also easily absorbed into the skin.

15 **Matrixyl** (palmitoly pentapeptide-3): this is a compound made up of combined peptides that helps prevent wrinkles forming and smooths out those already there. It can dramatically improve the appearance of skin, making it smoother, firmer and more refined. It can also boost collagen synthesis and encourage the skin to become plumper. A great ingredient and one we use in our own *X116 Anti-Wrinkle Cream*.

16 **MSM** (methylsulfonylmethane): a wonderfully soothing supplement that has a great effect on joint pain, eczema and dermatitis, and has powerful skin-boosting effects too. Good for lessening wrinkles and stretch marks; also helps repair the skin following sun damage.

17 **Niacinamide or Nicotinamide** (vitamin B3): reduces inflammation, soothes redness, improves the appearance of acne. It also appears to have anti-ageing properties.

18 **Panthenol** (vitamin B5): smooths the skin, pulls in moisture and can help repair the skin too. You may also find it in the form of calcium pantothenate.

19 **Rosa mosqueta** (rosehip) oil: studies show this oil produces a powerful regenerative action on the skin, reducing the appearance of wrinkles and scarring, evening out skin tone and colour, reducing sun damage and sunspots. It also has a superb effect on scarring so is very useful following surgery, once wounds have healed.

20 **SOD** (superoxide dismutase): another powerful antioxidant that has superb skin-protecting and rejuvenating powers.

21 **Tazarotene**: can reduce skin ageing and is a powerful rejuvenator. Currently only available on prescription in the UK.

22 **Vitamin A** (in naturally occurring forms such as retinol, retinaldehyde and retinyl palmitate): a powerful antioxidant with proven results for skin rejuvenation.

23 **Vitamin C**: this superb antioxidant can pack a powerful punch when applied on to your skin as well as when taken internally. It protects the skin from UVA damage, helps boost collagen synthesis and is a general all-round antioxidant superstar. Look for products that have 'stabilised vitamin C'. Ester-C is also a good choice as it's more easily absorbed by the skin.

24 **Vitamin E** (tocopherol or tocopherol acetate): another powerful antioxidant that can reduce sun damage and protect the skin. The most active form is alpha tocopherol.

25 **Vitamin K**: very helpful in reducing dark circles under the eyes, and helps tone down the reddened appearance of thread veins and spider veins. It's an important ingredient in our new *X119 Eye Gel*.

WHY NOT COLLAGEN?

Yes, it's true that many creams contain collagen. Yes, it's true that more collagen in our skin would be a good thing. However the problem is that collagen molecules are simply too large to be absorbed directly through the skin. So no matter how many you rub into your skin they will simply stay perched on top of your epidermis doing very little. Some new creams use cold, purportedly to shrink collagen molecules so they can be nudged into the skin. We are not convinced.

Make-up for your new face

It's easy to get caught in a time-warp when it comes to make-up. Too many women decide on a 'look' in their teens or early twenties, and then just stay with it for decades – or until they keel over and die! However there is nothing as dating and ageing as old-fashioned make-up. This is particularly true when you have undergone cosmetic surgery. After all, why not make the very best of your new face or features?

Our best advice is to go and get expert help. Most of the major cosmetic companies will give you a makeover, advising on the latest looks and what would best suit your features and skin. Choose a company whose products you like and go with an open mind, prepared to try out new ideas. You don't have to buy all the items – it's just a way of trying out new products and new looks. An alternative is to pay for a lesson by an independent make-up artist; it will cost more but you will be given advice on a broad range of products and makes. You will also be taught how to put on make-up and to get the effect you're looking for.

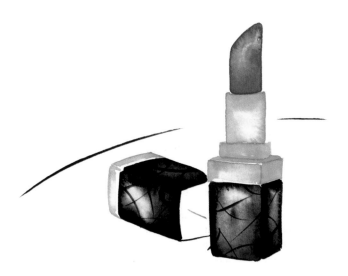

THE GOLDEN RULES FOR ANTI-AGEING MAKE-UP

- Choose your foundation carefully. Too much heavy foundation can be ageing as it will cling to wrinkles and furrows, making them more – not less – noticeable. Think light and dewy not caked-on. Aim for a light-textured foundation that matches your skin tone perfectly (test it on your jawline, not on the underside of your wrist, and always ask for help if you're not certain).

- There is no single rule about how to apply foundation. You can use a damp make-up sponge or dab it gently using your fingers. However, never pull or drag the skin.

- Powder is really only necessary and useful if you have very oily skin. Otherwise it can be rather ageing.

- If you have dry skin, it may be worth experimenting with a primer under your foundation.

- Concealers can work miracles, but go easy. Less is more. Light-diffusing concealers with yellow undertones will help to mask dark shadows under the eyes. Avoid very pale concealers – they should always match your skin tone. Apply your concealer after your foundation.

- A little blusher gives definition to cheekbones and imparts a healthy glow. Again, subtlety is the key. Be guided by the experts to a blusher that suits your natural skin tone. Suck in your cheeks to find your cheekbones and blend it in upwards and outwards towards your hairline. Make sure there are no obvious edges on show.

- Lips get thinner as we get older and can do with some help. Generally speaking, gloss lipstick makes lips look fuller than matt shades. A good lip liner can work miracles: learn how to draw a line just outside your natural lip contours to make lips look bigger. Then fill in with your lipstick, covering over the lip liner. Add a little bit of lip gloss in the centre of your lips. As always, choose lipstick colours that suit your skin tone. As you get older, mid-tones are kindest; very dark or very pale lipsticks can look ageing. Candy colours are best left to the kids.

- Mascara may be all you need on your eyes. Curl your eyelashes before applying (it really opens up your eyes). You don't have to spend a fortune on mascara but do replace it regularly, about every two months at the least. Black mascara is dramatic (and works well on olive and dark skins) but if you have paler skin you might try brown, or brownish-black as a less harsh alternative.

- Eyeshadow needs care. Leave the wild colours and outrageous looks to the seriously young and trendy. Softer neutrals are the kindest to older eyes. Opt for matt tones rather than shimmering sparkles which will emphasise wrinkles. Lighter shades open out the eyes.

- Eyeliner also requires a bit of thought. Yes, it can define and emphasise your eyes but make sure it's a soft look. Brown can be a gentler alternative to black. Eye pencils or even eyeshadow applied with an applicator can give a softer, smudgier look that opens up the eyes. If you like eyeliner but have a wobbly hand, consider permanent make-up.

- Don't forget your eyebrows. Not only do they need a good shape (see below) but you should also make sure they have a good colour. Professional dyeing is a great option or use an eyebrow pencil – or even a little mascara – to give definition. It's a marvellous way to open up your face.

EYEBROW SHAPING

We would really recommend you take a regular trip to the beauty salon to have your eyebrows shaped. If you've never had this done before, you could be in for a surprise. Shaping shaggy eyebrows can give as dramatic a change to your face as a facelift (well, nearly). As always, don't go too far. One of the natural signs of ageing is for our eyebrows to get thinner, so super-plucked eyebrows can add years to your look. Over-plucking also draws attention to sharp or severe features. So shape rather than shave. If you have overdone it, or if your eyebrows are naturally thinning as you get older, use a little subtle make-up to disguise the fact. Choose an eye pencil one shade lighter than your hair colour (overly dark eyebrows are simply too severe) and use it to balance your brows, gently stroking in a fuller shape. A good alternative is permanent make-up (see below).

While you're at the salon you might consider having both eyebrows and eyelashes dyed.

PERMANENT MAKE-UP

Imagine not having to bother with full make-up every day! While some women love spending hours in front of the mirror, others find it a bore and a waste of time. Still others never quite get the hang of applying make-up and always look a little over- or underdone (or even mis-done!). Permanent make-up is a revolutionary beauty treatment that is used to define your eyes, brows, lips and cheeks to give the perfect imitation of superbly applied make-up. We offer it at our Centre as the perfect finishing touch – and our patients are delighted with the results.

The effect is achieved by infusing hypoallergenic pigments into the dermal layer of your skin; it's a little like very subtle tattooing at a more superficial level.

It starts with a consultation to assess your colouring and face shape. Then the consultant will create your own unique look, initially with conventional cosmetics, so you can try out different approaches and tailor-make your ideal result. Once you have approved the design, it is fed into computerised equipment and the pigments are mixed. They are then injected into your skin. The results can be as subtle or as dramatic as you wish – though personally we would always advise a subtle natural look.

It's not painful. You could say it's akin to having your eyebrows plucked. A session usually lasts about forty minutes and you will go back for a follow-up treatment after about three to five weeks to allow any final adjustments to be made to the shape and colour. The results will usually last for several years.

- Eyes: permanent eye enhancement can create either a defined liner (great if you always end up with a wavering line when you try to apply eyeliner) or subtle shadow. It makes your eyes appear larger and more striking. This is superb for anyone who suffers from allergies to pollen or conventional make-up, and also those with contact lens sensitivities.

- Eyebrows: eyebrows give shape to the face yet many people have thin eyebrow hair or very pale hair. This technique is achieved by using fine hair by hair simulation or a subtle colour mist infusion.

- Cheeks: a very subtle glow to the cheeks can emphasise bone structure and give definition to your face shape. Perfect if you often feel washed out, or if you never quite get blusher right.

- Lips: defines your natural lip contours and gives a haze of colour across the lips. Gives a very smart, groomed look. You can easily apply lipstick or gloss over the top to change your look.

Hair

A great hairdresser can take years off you. There is nothing more ageing than a cut that doesn't flatter your face shape or a colour that saps all the life from your complexion.

TEN COMMON HAIR MISTAKES THAT ADD ON THE YEARS

1 Tight perms. Sorry, but they always spell granny. Keep curls soft and vary the size of rollers for a natural look.

2 Using half a can of hairspray. Stiff over-coiffed styles that don't move when you do are incredibly dated.

3 Keeping the same hairstyle you had ten, twenty, thirty years ago. Pins you to a decade at first glance.

4 Dragging your hair back tightly from your face – a very unforgiving look. Useful for teenagers and twenty-somethings who want to add years or gravitas; otherwise forget it.

5 Hair colour too far away from your natural skin tones; bleach blonde doesn't look girlish, it looks sad and aged if you're not a natural blonde. Raven locks will wash you out unless you have the skin tone that sits naturally with black hair. Warmer hair tones are kinder to older faces.

6 Scrunchies and bobbles. They're for little girls, not grown-ups. If you want to decorate your hair opt for subtle, sophisticated slides or a single sparkling diamond kirby-grip.

7 Plaits and bunches. Not a good look for anyone out of their teens. You look silly, not sophisticated.

8 Very severe geometric styles. Tough on older faces; you need a little softness to blunt the edges.

9 Very long hair. Looks odd and slightly mad on older women but you don't have to go for ultra-short either. Keep it above shoulder-level is a good rule of thumb for anyone over forty. If you can't bear the idea of cutting your hair, keep the back long (in a V shape) and have softer layers at the front.

10 Not bothering with conditioner. Hair gets drier as it gets older and you run the risk of ending up with coarse, wiry, Brillo pad locks. Always keep your hair in peak condition: sleek, glossy hair looks younger and feels gorgeous.

WHAT'S THE BEST CUT?

You need to pick the very best hair stylist you can afford – it's a real investment so don't be tempted to cut corners or save pennies. Take as much care in choosing your stylist as you would a surgeon; again, this is a relationship that will need to stand the test of time. Find someone who understands your hair, your face and what you want to achieve and you're well on the way to looking and feeling wonderful. It's worth bearing in mind that, just as your hair colour changes as you get older, so too does the shape of your face. Keeping the same style you had when you were young can be a big mistake: you need constant fine-tuning and tweaking to look your best.

It's fine to take in pictures of styles you like, but be guided by your stylist – they will be able to tell you if your preferred style will flatter you, or overpower you.

There might well be ways of tweaking it to give the same effect but with a more flattering look for you.

FACE SHAPE	BEST SHAPES	AVOID
Round	Go for styles that fall under the chin. A light fringe is good. Also layered cuts that sweep forward on to your cheeks. Wispy looks and tapered ends are softening.	Heavy bobs, blunt cuts and heavy fringes.
Square	Face-framing layers. Short spiky cuts. Long sleek styles with layers that start at the jaw and continue downwards.	Solid bobs (particularly chin-length ones). Thick solid fringes.
Heart-shaped	A light, textured fringe that can be swept to one side. Keep layers soft, long and wavy (ideally grazing your cheekbones).	Harsh geometric cuts. Thick solid fringes. Choppy layers.
Long	Create width with a solid fringe. Chin-length bobs and cuts create an illusion of width. Mid-length curls and waves also work well.	Short curls and all very short styles in general. Very long hair (if you must have long hair have it layered or keep it shorter at the front).
Oval	Medium to long layered cuts. Choose layers near your best feature – cheekbones, lips or chin.	Short layers that add height to the top of your head. Blunt cuts aren't great either.

WHICH COLOUR WOULD SUIT ME BEST?

You could go naturally grey, but we suspect that's unlikely. Grey and white hair is synonymous with ageing so most women prefer to retain their natural colour as they get older, or take the chance to improve on nature. Again, you'll need to spend money. It really is worth going to the best colourist you can possibly afford. Specialists will look at your skin tone and your hair and be able to advise you on the best possible choices. As you get older, your skin colour changes slightly: due to a lessening of pigment (melanin) in the skin it becomes lighter. So, generally speaking, as you get older, you will need a slightly (note the slightly) lighter hair colour than you had when you were very young.

Permanent colour is the easiest way of keeping your look for the longest time. Highlights, lowlights and weaves can give a richly textured look and will need less root maintenance than solid colour.

IF YOUR SKIN IS	TRY THESE COLOURS	AND AVOID THESE
Fair	Honey blonde, ash blonde, auburn	Very dark brown or black
Freckled	Warm reds, copper and auburn; dark blonde with golden tones	Bright blonde, dark brown, black
Rosy-tinged	Cooler ash blondes, brown, ash brown	Reds, auburn, golden blonde or golden browns
Sallow	Beige blonde, auburn, copper	Golden blonde, golden brown, dark brown or black
Olive	Rich auburn, mahogany, warm brown	Blonde (any kind), very bright copper, crimson, aubergine
Dark brown/black	Black, dark auburn; rich highlights in red, aubergine, mahogany	Blonde, copper, ash tones

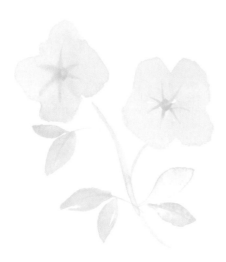

Yes, nails matter

Beautiful nails make a woman look well-groomed and 'finished'. Well-tended nails show you take care of yourself and pay attention to detail. Yet we can't count how many women look absolutely perfect until you notice their ragged nails. Keep your nails in tip-top condition by having regular manicures (and pedicures) or spend time giving yourself a DIY version at home. Don't be tempted by 'Footballers' Wives' long talons – they look common and rather ageing. Keep your nails reasonably short but perfectly shaped and in superb condition.

- Apply hand cream or oil every night before going to bed; put on a pair of cotton gloves to allow the cream or oil to sink in and really nourish your skin.

- Once a week, soak your hands and nails in warm enriching oil – olive, sweet almond or coconut are all very soothing and nourishing.

- Softly push back cuticles. Never cut cuticles.

- Use a professional tool to remove ridges and buff your nails.

- Then gently file your nails into shape. Never cut down the sides of your nails.

- Apply base or undercoat; it is worth spending the extra time as it helps give a smooth surface for your polish and will keep the colour for longer.

- You may want to apply a conditioner to strengthen and protect your nails.

- Choose a flattering shade of polish for your nails. For everyday wear softer, more neutral colours are best.

- Stroke on polish up the centre of your nail, from the base to the tip. Then work outwards to the sides. Always allow the first coat to dry completely before applying the second.

- Add a top coat for extra protection and gloss.

ARTIFICIAL NAILS

If your own nails are in an appalling state, if you simply cannot grow them or can't get out of the (unappealing) habit of biting them, you might want to consider artificial nails. They do look great – but be aware that they will require regular salon trips for maintenance and that they weaken your real nails. It can take several months for your nails to return to their original condition once they have had false nails, wraps or tips applied.

There are various types available.

- Acrylic nails: strong and long-lasting. In the hands of an experienced nail technician they are a good option but in less experienced hands they can appear thick and very obviously fake. You will need to have them filled every two to three weeks as your own nails grow. Infection is a danger with inexperienced technicians.

- Gel nails: a gel is applied and then set under UV light. These are more natural and less prone to infection in that air can still reach through the porous gel. You will need to wear gloves when using detergents and chemicals as these can also reach through the gel. Not as strong as acrylic nails; if you type a lot these might not be a good option.

- Sculptured nails: gel, fibreglass or acrylic is applied to your nails and then sculpted over foil or metal.

- Wraps: silk, linen or fibre wraps or tips are glued to the nail.

Take a hard look at your wardrobe

It's amazing how many women simply don't know how to dress. We're not being rude but, truly, so many women simply have no concept of style or how to flatter their shape with clothes.

THE TOP TEN CLASSIC MISTAKES

1 Shapeless clothes. Yes, it's tempting to hide inside voluminous trousers, or even a floor-length kaftan. But truly, baggy clothes do you no favours: they simply hang off the largest part of your body (be it breasts, stomach, hips or thighs) and make your whole body look as large as the plump bits.

2 Staying stuck in a time-warp. You know the story: shoulder-pads, puffed sleeves, sloppy Joes, sky-high stilettos. Wearing the same styles you wore when you were younger is a hideous mistake, ageing you immediately.

3 Wearing the 'uniform' for your age. Nowhere is it written in stone that once you hit a certain age you have to swap stylish clothes for slacks, turtle necks, tan tights and elastic-waisted skirts. Naturally you don't want to look like mutton dressed as lamb, but keep your look subtly updated. Can seventy-somethings wear jeans? Of course – if they have the right shape.

4 Ignoring your shape. Look in the mirror: is your outfit flattering? Does it suit you? Does it draw attention to your good bits and tone down the bad bits? It's incredible how few women actually shop according to their shape.

5 Blindly following fashion. This follows on from number four. So many women will buy clothes simply because they are fashionable, with total disregard as to whether they actually suit their shape and age. Always stick to clothes that flatter your shape – add high fashion detailing with accessories if necessary.

6 Black, black, black. Nothing wrong with black – it's sexy, chic and slimming. But keep it sharp and make it interesting with really fabulous accessories and maybe the odd splash of colour, or it becomes a bland uniform.

7 Clothes that are the wrong size. Too big or too small, both are fashion crimes. You need clothes that really fit. Fitted clothes can take years, and pounds, off the way you look.

8 The wrong colours. Some colours lift your skin tone and make you look bright, fresh and gorgeous. Others will make you look ten years older. If you're unsure about which colour and tones really suit you, a colour consultation can be enlightening. You're swathed with different-coloured scarves according to your 'season' – everyone is either spring, summer, autumn or winter (according to skin tone, eye and hair colour). It sounds pretty insane but it can be a real eye-opener.

9 Awful underwear. A well-fitting bra and the right pants can make an unbelievable difference. Have yourself fitted for your bra by an expert. Pick your underwear according to your outfit. Subtle support-wear can tuck in a protruding tummy or slice a few millimetres off your thighs.

10 Inappropriate clothes. Your wardrobe needs to be your ally, not your worst enemy. Clothes give out messages, so make sure you mean what you're saying. If you're in business the right outfit can make or break a deal. If you're looking for a date, you might be putting off the people you want to attract by giving out the wrong signals. If you aren't confident with your clothes choices, most big stores now have personal shoppers who can advise you.

DRESSING FOR YOUR SHAPE: THE FASHION RULES

Large breasts

The main problem here is looking top-heavy so you want to avoid anything that provides a block of solid colour over your top half.

- Choose wide open necklines or deep V-necks.
- Smartly tailored jackets, coats and dresses will look good if you pick the right shape. Go for single-breasted jackets with a nipped-in waist and deep V-neck.
- Tailored shirts are fine but make sure they fit properly and don't gape.
- Fine knits are more flattering; silky mixes won't cling so much. Choose soft cardigans and wraps rather than sweaters.
- Wrap tops and dresses are very forgiving to large breasts.
- Forget about high-neck tops and polo-neck jumpers.
- Avoid double-breasted jackets, Nehru collars and jackets that button right up to the neck.
- Steer clear of thick, heavy knits.
- Avoid large bright patterns on your top half. A patterned skirt, however, can draw attention away from your top.

Large stomach

Clever dressing can disguise a large tummy.

- Choose tops that gently roll over the stomach area. Ruching can be very flattering.
- Never tuck tops in. Never choose overly short tops. Deep V-necks are a good look.
- Jackets, nipped in at the waist (but undone) give the illusion of a trim waist.
- If you have slim hips draw attention here with a low-slung belt.
- Cardigans in fine slinky knits with asymmetrical hemlines confuse the eye and draw attention away from the waist.
- Long-line tailored jackets and frock coats look elegant and disguise a large tum.
- Dresses in floaty, delicate printed fabrics distract the eye away from the stomach.
- Empire lines and soft smock styles are a great friend in need.
- Flat-fronted trousers are forgiving. Avoid elasticated waists and either very high waists or very low-rise (your stomach will hang over the top).
- Long slinky scarves can discreetly hide extra inches.
- Steer clear of double-breasted coats and jackets.
- Avoid belted coats – and belts around the waist in general.

Pear shape

- Draw attention to your slim top half with fitted tops and nipped-in waists. Slash and boat necks are flattering.

- Keep skirts A-line or gently flaring. Avoid clingy materials and bias cuts that will hug your hips and bond with your thighs.

- Jackets need to be long-line, preferably three-quarter length with a nipped-in waist and large lapels. Severely cropped is another option as it emphasises the waist. Otherwise always well below the hip. Never ever on the hips themselves.

- Wear a gorgeous belt nipped in around your waist.

- Skirts and dresses will always be more flattering than trousers.

- If you must wear trousers keep to palazzo pants or wide-legged boot-cut styles.

- Sorry, but jeans will never be a great look for you; if you must, keep them flared, plain and very dark indigo or black.

- Wrap tops and dresses are a disaster, dragging the eye inexorably to your hips and bum.

- Stick to dark colours on the bottom half – they're more flattering.

- Wear bright colours or wild prints on your top half to draw the eye up. Interesting necklaces and jazzy earrings can help too.

Short

- Palazzo pants and wide flares (worn with heels) look elegant and lengthen your shape. Wear with tops the same colour.

- Dresses worn over trousers add height.

- Very long skirts are elegant and you can wear high heels.

- Slim jeans tucked into knee-high boots look lean and sexy.

- Calf-length skirts and tops in the same colour elongate the body. Add a gorgeous slim belt for interest at the waist.

- Forget cropped trousers and pedal-pushers.

- Skinny jeans look good with heels and are much more flattering than bootcuts for you (unless you're plump).

- Long-line jackets that end on the thigh or three-quarter-length coats and jackets.

- Very long coats will swamp you.

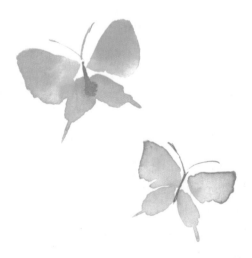

The importance of good posture

Posture can totally change the way you look, and also the way you feel. Simple adjustments to the way you stand can add inches to your height and several cup sizes to the appearance of your breasts. Your stomach will tuck in, trimming off inches, when you hold yourself properly. Even your buttocks can appear more pert. Not only will you look better, you'll also feel better. Psychologists have found that a stooped, slumped posture encourages depression, while an upright position encourages the production of endorphins, the feelgood chemicals. All the nerve pathways that leave the brain eventually go through muscles, so there is a definite connection between what we think and what we experience.

Children possess perfect poise and a free and easy posture; they're divinely fluid and balanced. But, as we get older, life takes its toll and we start to lose that ease of movement. In particular, if we are unhappy with a specific part of our body, it is common unconsciously to try to hide it, hence the hunching of shoulders to hide breasts that are considered too small or too large.

Following cosmetic surgery you may find that your body starts to feel odd, as you adapt to having more or less body to feel! If you haven't had posture training before (and we would hope you have), you absolutely must have some now. You will need to learn how to hold yourself so you show your new body or face off to its best advantage.

Basic good posture involves having your body in the best possible alignment, with back and abdominal muscles equally strong and the spine in the optimum position.

Unfortunately, it's really hard to teach yourself good posture because, with the best will in the world, you can't see yourself from the outside in. You may think you're totally straight but ten to one you'll be at quite a tilt. This is where it makes great good sense to call in the master posture experts. Alexander Technique and the Feldenkrais Method are both superb for putting your brand-new body into perfect alignment. Pilates and yoga can help, and many personal trainers now take additional courses in postural alignment and correctional exercise (such as our own Scott Bryant who uses the superb C.H.E.K. System of exercise and postural alignment).

ALEXANDER TECHNIQUE

A straightforward, down-to-earth technique that really can make you look taller and slimmer. It can also help silence stress and banish the blues, give you significant relief from back and neck pain and ease the ache of arthritis.

The technique was developed by Frederick Mathias Alexander, an Australian actor who wanted to find out why he was losing his voice. He closely analysed his movements and discovered that he was pulling his head back and down on to his spine with an enormous amount of tension. The tension was impairing his breathing and causing constriction of the larynx. Alexander began to experiment and finally came up with a solution for the tension. He went on to develop an entire system which would enable almost anyone to return to the comfort and ease they enjoyed as babies and small children. Many people appear to 'grow' with AT by as much as an inch and a half (they are actually straightening up); and they appear to lose weight at the same time. Because we have a tendency to sink down into our hips, by allowing a lengthening of the torso a redistribution of fat tissue takes place and you can easily become taller and thinner.

The technique is usually taught in individual lessons or small classes. Your teacher will painstakingly observe how you use your body, whether standing, sitting or walking. Then they will teach you how subtly to change your patterns of movement to restore your body to its natural balance. Don't expect miracles overnight – a basic course will consist of around thirty lessons and many people go on to take many more.

It takes hard work and dedication for the best results and you will be expected to practise every day. But it's worth it.

FELDENKRAIS METHOD

The Feldenkrais Method was developed by Moshe Feldenkrais who was born in Russia and gained a PhD in engineering and physics. He noted that most people are quite unaware of how they hold their bodies, which parts move easily and which are stilted or lacking in mobility. By gently moving the person's body in unfamiliar ways, Feldenkrais found people could become more aware of how their bodies moved and could actually alter the neuromuscular patterns that organise and control movement. The result was freedom from pain and increased flexibility.

The Feldenkrais Method is taught in two distinct ways. One-to-one sessions are known as Functional Integration and comprise manipulation, generally carried out on a low couch. It's all very gentle, minimal and pleasant. You will frequently be asked to 'check in' with your body, noticing sensations and getting in touch with how you feel. You will also be taught how to perform the minute movements for yourself. A lot of visualisation is involved, to help your body make the right moves. Alternatively you can learn the Method via Awareness through Movement classes and workshops in which small groups carry out gentle exercises guided by a teacher. Many of the movements taught in class are drawn directly from babyhood and childhood so you're quite likely to find yourself rolling or twisting on the floor just like a toddler. Great fun.

NOTE: Pilates, yoga, t'ai chi and qi gong will also help your posture enormously. If you get the chance, do check out these great exercise systems.

TOP TIPS FOR BETTER POSTURE

Standing

1 Stand straight. Stop slouching on one side: think about standing on both feet equally. Feel your toes spreading to hold your weight. Imagine you have a string in the centre of your head that gently pulls you up.

2 Tuck your bottom in and pull in your belly button to your spine, so you are using your core muscles like a girdle to hold yourself. That gives a good basis for the lower back.

3 Most of us poke our chins out too far. The head should be balanced with the chin tucked in.

Walking

1 Take even strides. Some people pull themselves along, over-using their hamstrings; others lean forwards and over-stride. The most sensible walk is one that uses easy, even strides.

2 Keep your balance. We are designed to balance on one leg after the other.

3 Walk low. High heels can throw the pelvis forward which, in turn, will throw the whole body out of alignment. Eventually it can cause shortening in some muscles which could lead to back pain. Obviously low heels are the best for your posture, but that's not always possible. If you need to be in heels for part of your day, just make sure you wear flats for the rest.

Sitting at work

1 Choose your chair with care. Ideally you should sit with your knees lower than your pelvis. Your seat should be high enough for you to be able to relax your shoulders, leaving your arms at a 90-degree angle to your desk. If the chair has arms they should be low enough to fit under your desk.

2 Position your computer high. If you work on screen your computer should be on a stand rather than on the desk (yes, even your laptop), so that you can look directly at it, rather than down at it. Equally, make sure it is directly in front of you rather than situated to one side.

Sitting at home

1 Choose firm support. It's tempting to slouch on the sofa but it's the worst possible position for your back. You should have a reasonably firm support behind you so pick a more upright chair or protect your back with a pile of firm cushions.

2 Keep straight. Your eyes lead your head which, in turn, leads the whole body. If you're watching TV you should be directly facing it with your head balanced. If you're reading a book, lift the book up towards you rather than bending over your lap.

Driving

1 A small wedge or lumbar roll to support the lower back can provide considerable relief for many drivers.

2 Teachers of the Alexander Technique often suggest you put a large paperback under your bottom when driving to place your spine into a better position.

3 Take regular breaks and stand up and stretch to readjust your body. Any kind of travelling is uncomfortable for the body because you are cramped in one position for a considerable time. You have to try to keep moving and not get stuck in one position for too long.

EXERCISES TO HELP YOUR POSTURE

1 Teachers of the Alexander Technique recommend you lie on the floor for between fifteen and twenty minutes during the day with your head balanced on a small pile of paperback books (about the same height as your hand span). Gently roll on to the books and bring your feet in towards your buttocks so your knees point towards the ceiling. Hands should be gently resting on either side of your navel.

Try to become aware of any tension in your body and, as you feel it, don't try to correct your position, just think about your spine lengthening and the tension disappearing.

This exercise can replace the fluid between the discs of our spine and add an inch or more to your height during the day.

2 Before you settle down to work you should aim to run through the following. Stand straight with your weight distributed evenly, your stomach and bottom held in and your shoulders back. Turn your head gently to the left and then to the right (five times each side).

Move your left ear down to your left shoulder then repeat on the other side (x 5).

Raise both shoulders up towards your ears and down again, breathing in on the way up and out on the way down (x 5).

With your left hand on your left shoulder and your right hand on your right shoulder, bring your elbows together in front and circle backwards (x 5).

Place your knuckles in your back and gently stretch backwards.

You can practise these exercises whenever you have a few spare minutes – they are equally effective in a sitting position.

Your smile: Cosmetic Dentistry

Going to the dentist used to be something most people dreaded. Not for nothing do we have the phrase 'it was like pulling teeth'! But now it's a vital part of the rejuvenation package. It's all well and good having a perfect face but not so good if the whole effect is ruined the moment you open your mouth. Snaggle teeth, huge gaps and discoloured incisors aren't a good look so it's no surprise that cosmetic dentistry is now a boom business in the UK. It's taken a while to catch on though. In the past we tended to fight shy of having our teeth 'fixed', put off (with good reason) by the sight of all those Hollywood gleaming tombstones. Just as a facelift should look totally natural, so should your teeth. If teeth are too big, too bright, too plumb-line straight, they look unnatural and draw attention (for all the wrong reasons).

Fortunately balance is returning to cosmetic dentistry and even Hollywood is now queuing up for the 'European look' – teeth that look fresh and bright with pleasing shapes. You need people to compliment you on your gorgeous smile, rather than have them asking what you've had done to your teeth. As with all forms of cosmetic surgery, self-esteem and confidence are key. Vast numbers of people go through life ashamed of their teeth. We have seen people who mumble or even hold their hands over their mouths to hide their teeth. Sorting out problem teeth can be a revelation, giving back the confidence to talk freely and smile and laugh as widely as you like.

We find a lot of our patients automatically have cosmetic dentistry following a facelift or other work on the face. It's the finishing touch. The good news is that the vast majority of dental work is actually pretty non-invasive. Most dental problems can be fixed by relatively simple and painless procedures such as whitening and veneers.

WHITENING

Everyone wants lovely white clean teeth because they look young and pleasing. The colour of your teeth is determined by your DNA, just like the colour of your eyes and length of your nose. Some of us are blessed with gorgeous white teeth, others draw the short straw and are doomed to naturally yellow or dull teeth. However nature catches up even with the genetically lucky ones and, as we get older, the dentine (the soft pulpy substance that lies beneath the enamel and which protects the nerves and blood vessels of the tooth) starts to change colour, becoming more yellow. With the best will in the world, no whitening toothpaste will be able to deal with that. Our everyday diet also takes its toll on the teeth: think of the stains left in your tea or coffee cup, think how a strong curry can mark a plate – no wonder our teeth get stained.

Whitening toothpastes mainly work because they contain mild abrasives that help to keep your teeth white by removing any stains. They are certainly useful but if you really want a more dramatic improvement you will need to see a dentist for professional whitening. Whitening will not make a complete colour change (you would need a veneer for that) but it will lighten the existing shade quite considerably. It may be tempting to try one of the 'at-home' whitening kits that are now readily available, but we'd not recommend it. Whitening requires a specially made tray that fits into your mouth like a gum shield while DIY kits use a one-size-fits-all tray which really isn't advisable.

Your cosmetic dentist will check your teeth and make sure your gums are healthy. Bleaching may not be recommended if you have gum disease or crowns. Then they will take impressions of your teeth – both upper and lower sets – using a tray and dental putty. From these impressions a plastic sleeve will be made that fits precisely and snugly around your teeth. A small amount of bleaching gel (the active ingredient is usually hydrogen peroxide or carbamide peroxide) is then inserted into the sleeve and placed over your teeth for between thirty minutes and one hour. As the active ingredient is broken down, oxygen gets into the enamel of the tooth, lightening it. You will be taught how to carry out the procedure yourself so you can continue with applications at home. The whole process takes between two to four weeks and you will have to apply the bleaching product once a day.

Some dentists prefer new products which can be applied for up to eight hours at a time, achieving good results within a week.

There is also a technique known as laser whitening, or power whitening, during which a laser is shone on the teeth to activate and speed up the chemical reaction. The procedure takes about an hour but is much more expensive than traditional whitening.

How white should you go? As always subtlety is the key. Having your teeth whitened is one of the easiest ways of making you look younger but you don't want people to put on sunglasses when they talk to you. The rule of thumb is never go lighter than the whites of your eyes. Why? When someone looks at you, their gaze flickers between your eyes and your mouth – if one overpowers the other, it looks weird and unnatural.

Cost? Low.

VENEERS

Porcelain veneers are probably the most commonly used procedure in cosmetic dentistry and can have dramatic results. They can be used to close up unsightly gaps in the teeth, or to align crowded or protruding teeth. They can also repair chips and cracks in the teeth and cover up staining. Unlike a crown, a veneer is wafer-thin.

Your dentist will take an impression of your teeth and then the veneer is made in a laboratory by a dental technician. Most veneers are made of porcelain although some are constructed of a natural colour composite material. Porcelain veneers take longer to produce but also last for a very long time (around ten to fifteen years on average). The benefit of composites, on the other hand, is that they can be completed in one visit although they are slightly more prone to staining than porcelain veneers and do tend to have a shorter life (around five to seven years). However, they can easily be replaced as necessary.

Some dentists market veneers (sometimes in combination with the fitting of bridges and implants) as a 'Dental Face Lift' or 'Smile Lift' – and it's easy to see why. The combination can totally transform your mouth and smile; it may be expensive but it's a great investment in your looks as the results can be breathtaking.

Cost? High.

CROWNS (CAPS)

You're probably familiar with crowns, a simple way of covering broken or heavily filled teeth. The tooth is filed down to a stump and then a false covering is adhered to the remains of the tooth. Sometimes crowns are combined with a bridge to fill a gap: the teeth either side of the gap are filed down and a crown is put right across, giving the impression of an unbroken line of perfect teeth.

Cost? Low (up to two crowns).

IMPLANTS

An alternative to bridgework to solve the problem of missing teeth. Implants are false teeth that are actually anchored to the bone. A titanium stud is inserted into the jaw (under either local or general anaesthetic). You should expect some discomfort and the stitches will need to stay in for up to ten days, which can feel uncomfortable. Your own bone fuses around the stud (this is known as osseointegration and takes between three to six months). Once the process is completed, a titanium post is screwed into the stud and finally the false tooth is fixed into it. It's a time-consuming and expensive procedure but results can be very good (providing your bone is in good condition).

Cost? Low (per tooth).

ORTHODONTICS (TEETH STRAIGHTENING)

You don't need to be a child to get yourself a mouthful of wire. Anybody of any age can benefit, it's just that it might take a little longer as you get older to see results.

This is a good option if your teeth really are in a jumble or if your jaw is incorrectly aligned. It's a long-term commitment: it can take up to two years to persuade teeth to behave themselves. The dentist (usually a specialist in this work, known as an orthodontist) will take X-rays of your teeth and plaster models of both jaws. Surgery may be necessary to correct the position of your jaw. Equally, some teeth may be extracted to create space for a balanced smile.

Crooked teeth are slowly pulled back into position with the use of a brace. Badly shaped or chipped teeth will be veneered to give an even look. It's expensive, time-consuming and can also involve a fair amount of discomfort, aching and even pain. However the results can be fabulous.

Cost? Medium to high.

GUM LIFTS/GRAFTS AND CONTOURING

These techniques are used to treat a gummy smile or build up areas of receding gum. Grafting takes tissue from one section of the mouth (usually the roof) and stitches it into the receding gum. It can be effective but your gums must be in good health for it to be carried out. It can be quite sore and is usually carried out under IV sedation. You have to use rinses before and after the procedure to keep the area free from infection. Gums will also continue to shrink with time and so the results cannot be permanent – you will probably need more treatment in about ten years.

Cost? Low to medium.

Contouring, on the other hand, is far less invasive and is usually permanent; it involves trimming and reshaping the gums (usually with a laser).

Cost? Low.

HOW TO FIND A GOOD COSMETIC DENTIST

You need to be just as careful choosing your cosmetic dentist as you do picking your surgeon. Over 80 per cent of dentists now offer cosmetic procedures (they are a highly lucrative part of their business) and any qualified dentist can offer cosmetic dentistry. There is no specific qualification or required training. However, as with all cosmetic work, the more experienced and knowledgeable your dentist, the better the results will be.

- Ask for recommendations: if you know anyone who has lovely teeth (and has had work done), word of mouth is always a good way to go. Your cosmetic surgeon or GP may also know good practitioners.

- The British Academy of Cosmetic Dentistry (BACD, see Resources) holds a register of cosmetic dentists who have carried out fifty hours of post-graduate education in cosmetic dentistry within the past two years.

- Check websites of dentists you are considering and ask for their brochures. Pick practices that focus on cosmetic dentistry every day.

- Choose two or three you feel might be right for you and arrange consultations.

- Check that the dentists you are considering are experienced in the procedure you require and are up to date with the latest techniques.

- At your consultation ask to see before and after photographs of people who have had the same procedure you are seeking. You might also ask to speak to them.

- Many dentists offer computer imaging to simulate the planned changes. This gives you the chance to see how your mouth would look, and also to fine-tune exactly what you want. 3-D mock-ups can also be made, which are really useful.

- Make sure you feel comfortable and confident with your dentist. Your gut instinct counts for a lot. If you don't feel confident, look elsewhere.

TOP TEN TIPS FOR A BEAUTIFUL SMILE

1 Brush your teeth twice a day – without fail.

2 Floss at least once a day.

3 Clean your tongue with a tongue scraper or toothbrush daily to keep your breath fresh.

4 Rinse daily with a mouthwash to help keep your gums healthy.

5 Keep your intake of sugary and acidic foods low. If you do have a sugary snack, chew sugar-free gum or have a small piece of cheese to help prevent the sugar attacking your teeth.

6 Don't brush immediately after eating fruit or acidic foods – you could damage the enamel. Wait half an hour.

7 Keep your intake of red wine and black coffee low to keep teeth bright.

8 Visit your dentist twice a year and have a professional clean-up by your dentist or hygienist twice yearly too.

9 Change your toothbrush (or brush head) regularly – as soon as the bristles start to splay out.

10 Never use your teeth for opening bottles or biting hard materials.

Enjoy your life!

We sincerely hope you have found this book useful and interesting. We would also hope that you will take the time and effort to try out what we suggest. Truly, we know it works – we have seen incredible results time and time again. Thousands of women can't be wrong!

Taking charge of your health and beauty can be incredibly liberating. Shifting your diet, getting into an exercise regime, taking supplements are all totally natural ways to make you look – and feel – years younger and miles better. Adding some cosmetic procedures simply takes the process a little further, makes you that little bit more beautiful.

Life is for living. Don't wait for changes to happen – make them happen. Take charge of yourself, your looks and we guarantee you will be stunned at how good you feel. Don't ever think, I'm not worth it, or think stunning looks and a wonderful figure are only for the rich and famous. Absolutely not. Every woman is worth it. Every woman can look gorgeous. If it takes a little injection here or a small incision there, so be it. In the brave new world of cosmetic surgery almost anything is possible. So, throw off your preconceptions and prejudices – it's time to enjoy life!

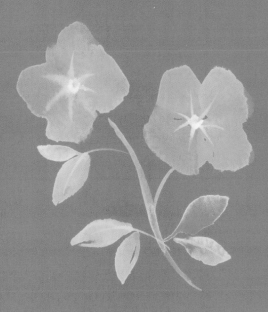

Resources

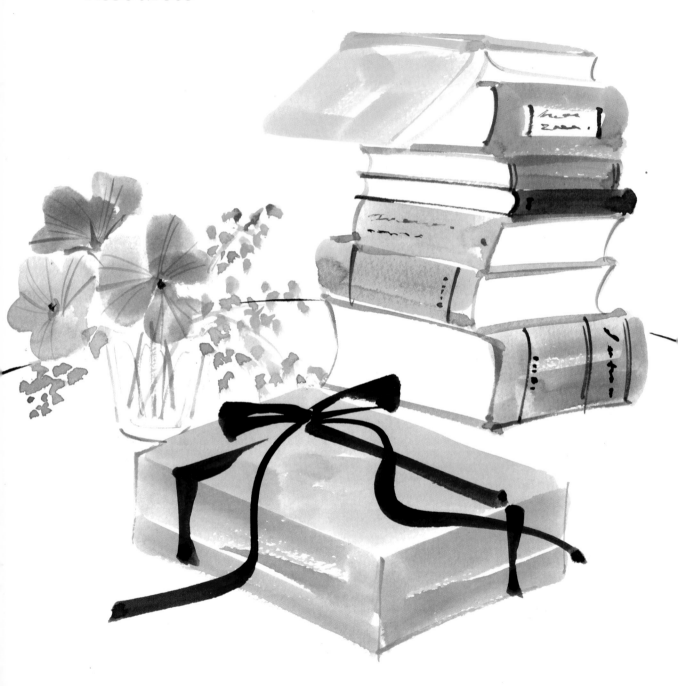

Dr Maurizio Viel
and Dr Roberto Viel
London Centre
for Aesthetic Surgery,
15 Harley Street,
London W1G 9QQ
020 7636 4272
www.lcas.com

We also hold clinics in Dublin,
Cardiff and Edinburgh.

Our skincare range
We have produced a small
range of skincare products that
we feel can truly help your
skin. For full information and
mail order details see our
website www.lcas.com
Or call 020 7636 4272

Our personal trainer
We often refer patients to our
personal trainer Scott Bryant.
Scott is a C.H.E.K. practitioner
specialising in corrective
exercise, nutrition and high
performance coaching. He is
based in London – for more
information see his website
www.activebryantsystems.com

Resources
British Association of Aesthetic
Plastic Surgeons (BAAPS)
Royal College of Surgeons,
35-43 Lincoln's Inn Fields
London WC2A 3PE
020 7405 2234
www.baaps.org.uk

British Association of
Plastic Surgeons (BAPS)
Royal College of Surgeons,
35-43 Lincoln's Inn Fields
London WC2A 3PE
www.baps.co.uk

British Association
of Dermatologists
4 Fitzroy Square
London W1T 5HQ
020 7383 0266
www.bad.org.uk

The Healthcare Commission
Finsbury Tower, 103-105
Bunhill Row
London EC1Y 8TG
0845 601 3012
www.healthcarecommission.org.uk

Hospitals, clinics and salons
offering invasive cosmetic
surgery and laser treatment
must be registered with the
Healthcare Commission. They
also handle complaints against
member clinics. Their website
offers advice and information
on procedures.

Department of Health
Richmond House, Whitehall
London SW1A 2NL
www.dh.gov.uk
General information on
cosmetic surgery. Downloads,
booklets and fact sheets for
various procedures. Provide
up-to-date warnings and advice

The General Medical Council
Regent's Place,
350 Euston Road,
London NW1 3JN
020 7915 3630
www.gmc-uk.org
Holds a list of surgeons on the
Specialist Register. Note: doctors
who started practising as
cosmetic surgeons before April
2002 may not be on the register.
Also handles complaints against
particular doctors.

The Independent Healthcare
Forum
Centre Point,
103 New Oxford Street,
London WC1A 1DU.
020 7379 8598
www.ihf.org.uk
A guide to the standards that
cosmetic surgeons should meet.
Also has a code of practice for
handling complaints.

Medicines and Healthcare
Products Regulatory Agency
(MHRA)
4/1 CO2 Market Towers
1 Nine Elms Lane
London SW8 5NQ
020 7084 3077
www.mhra.gov.uk
Up-to-the-minute information
on implants. Handles
complaints about medicines,
medical devices, treatments and
implants.

Advertising Standards
Authority,
Mid City Place,
71 High Holborn,
London WC1V 6QT
020 7492 2222
www.asa.org.uk
Handles complaints about
misleading or offensive
advertising; also stops direct
mail from companies (whether
sent by post, fax, text or email).

Breast Implant Information
Society (BIIS)
Highway Farm, Horsley Road,
Cobham
Surrey KT11 3JZ
07041 471225
www.biis.org

British Academy of
Cosmetic Dentistry (BACD)
29 Harley Street
London W1G 9QR
020 7612 4166
www.bacd.com

NHS Smoking Helpline
0800 169 0169
(7am – 11pm daily)
www.givingupsmoking.co.uk

Quitline
0800 00 2200
(9am – 9pm daily)
www.quit.org.uk
Individual, confidential advice
on giving up smoking.

Nutritional Therapy
The Institute for Optimum
Nutrition
Avalon House
Lower Mortlake Road
Richmond, Surrey
TW9 2JY
0870 979 1122
www.ion.ac.uk

National Register of
Personal Trainers
PO Box 3455
Marlow
Buckinghamshire
SL7 1WG
0870 200 6010
www.nrpt.co.uk

The C.H.E.K. Institute
www.chekinstitute.com
Holds a register of CHEK
practitioners in the UK and
other countries.

The British Wheel of Yoga
25 Jermyn Street
Sleaford, Lincolnshire
NG34 7RU
01529 306851
www.bwy.org.uk

National Institute of
Medical Herbalists
Elm House,
54 Mary Arches Street
Exeter, Devon
EX4 3BA
01392 426022
www.nimh.org.uk

Society of Homeopaths
11 Brookfield, Duncan Close
Moulton Park, Northampton
NN3 6WL
0845 450 6611
www.homeopathy-soh.org

Society of Teachers of the
Alexander Technique
1st Floor, Linton House
39-51 Highgate Road
London NW5 1RS
0845 230 7828
www.stat.org.uk

The Feldenkrais Guild
07000 785 506
www.feldenkrais.co.uk

T'ai chi Finder
www.taichifinder.co.uk
A web service that lists teachers
of t'ai chi and qi gong around
the UK.

Body Control Pilates
6 Langley Street
London WC2H 9JA
020 7379 3734
www.bodycontrol.co.uk

Permanent make-up
Natural Enhancement
26b Cambridge Road North
Chiswick, London
W4 4AA
0844 800 0397
www.naturalenhancement.co.uk

Index